TUBERCULOSIS
treated by
HOMOEOPATHY

TUBERCULOSIS *treated by* HOMOEOPATHY

Dr Rajeev Saxena

DCE, PhD, DBMS, [Gold Medallist] (VU)

Author of
A Study of Sarcodes, A Phenomenological Study of Nosodes, Understanding Glands, Endocrinology, The Homoeopathic Approach, Scientific Myology and Scientific Similimum, Homoeopathic Direct Energy, Medicines, Homoeopathic Hematology, Homoeopathy in Orthopaedics, Depression Treated by Bach Flower Therapy, A Scientific Study of Potency, Infections Treated by Homoeopathy, Aayush Nidan (Hindi), A Practical Guide to Thermoregulations, Classicals of Homoeopathy and Parkinson's Disease

New Central Book Agency (P) Ltd

LONDON

DELHI KOLKATA PUNE HYDERABAD ERNAKULAM

REGD. OFFICE

8/1 Chintamoni Das Lane, Kolkata 700 009, India
email: ncbapvtltd@eth.net

OVERSEAS

27 Catherine Court, Chase Road, Southgate, London, N14 4RB

EXPORT

212 Shahpur Jat, New Delhi 110 049
email: ncbaexp@ncbapvtltd.com

BRANCHES

4262/3 1st Floor, Flat Nos. 105 & 106
Ansari Road, Daryaganj, New Delhi 110 002
email: ncbadel@ncbapvtltd.com

House No. 3-1-315, 1st Floor
Nimboliadda, Kachiguda, Hyderabad 500 027
email: ncbahydb@ncbapvtltd.com

Shop Nos. 3 & 4, Vinayak Towers
681/B Budhwar Peth, Appa Balwant Chowk
Pune 411 002
email: ncbapune@ncbapvtltd.com

GSS Shopping Complex, 1st Floor
Opposite College Post Office, Convent Road
Ernakulam 682 035
email: ncbaernk@ncbapvtltd.com

TUBERCULOSIS TREATED BY HOMOEOPATHY

First Published: 2006, Reprinted: August 2009

PUBLISHER

New Central Book Agency (P) Ltd
8/1 Chintamoni Das Lane, Kolkata 700 009

TYPESETTER

Laser-O-Print

PRINTER

New Central Book Agency (P) Ltd
Web-Offset Division, Dhulagarh, Sankrail, Howrah

COVER DESIGNER

Soumen Paul

COVER PRINTER

Biswanath Studio
3 Garanhatta Street, Kolkata 700 006

TECHNICAL EDITOR

Dr Mita Sen, MBBS

PROJECT COORDINATORS

Prabhat Jas, Subas Maitra

ISBN: 81-7381-492-9

Price: Rs 135.00 [Rupees One Hundred and Thirty-five]

This work is
dedicated
to
Godess Harsidhdhi Devi Ma
of
Ujjain
and
Dr. M. K. Saxena, renowned homoeopathist,
Smt Nishibala Saxena and
Late Smt Raj Saxena
and Shree Girish Chandra Saxena
who have done everything for me
and my homoeopathy

Preface

Tuberculosis is a most dreaded disease of humanity. Though it can be controlled in a better way nowadays, yet its terrific effects on individual and society are long-lasting. The situation is more serious in developing countries and specially in India. It claims the majority of deaths.

The purpose in writing this work has been to present to the homoeopathic fraternity the subject of the disease along with its treatment. Modern chemotherapeutic medication (and vaccination) are there to check, treat and cure the tuberculosis, but the homoeopathic approach of treatment is gentle, easy, rapid and permanent. The poor communities, where this disease exists, need homoeopathy more than other systems, and the reason of this acute demand is very simple and sober. On one hand, homoeopathy which is a very specific way of therapeutics offers a complete treatment economically, on the other hand, its working style is easy, simple, non-violent and affordable.

Many chronic diseases have been successfully cured in homoeopathy and so is tuberculosis. Nearly every aspect important for homoeopathic philosophy and posological theories of tuberculosis has been presented herein in a simple language and lucid.

The author feels that this work is not only an indispensable tool for physicians and homoeopathic scientists but also to students and lay lovers of homoeopathy. This work provides readers the basics—the foundation of subject.

The author is highly grateful to all those authorities whose reference has been given in the bibliography. I am very much grateful to Shree Amitabha Sen Director, New Central Book Agency, who is publishing this work. Shree Sen has encouraged me to do such a serious work for cause of homoeopathy and, for that I am obliged to him very much.

I am also very thankful to my family members who have cooperated with me and stood by my side during preparation of this work. I am thankful to Smt. Sarla Saxena, my mother, Smt Taruna, my wife and master Yash, my son, and Sanjeev, Atul and Vinay who have given me moral support to complete this work. Vivek, Shubh, Shailee, Deepak, Preeti, Ruchi, Bhanu, Vidajee, Abhay, Amit, Kalpana, Kalesh and Animesh Mukherjee, these all my companions, have given me continuous encouragement.

I am also very much grateful to the erudite teachers of colleges and other institutions, the lay-readers and students, who have accepted and appreciated my works on homoeopathic medical science.

Finally, I would like to say that if this work proves its utility in treating and curing Tuberculosis – one of the most dreaded discase, I will feel my labour amply rewarded.

In name of God, Humble

16/6/2005
'Utsav'-A-37
Indrapuri Sethinagar
Ujjain (M. P.)
India

Rajeev Saxena

Contents

1 TUBERCULOSIS : A HISTORICAL REVIEW

Tuberculosis is an infection caused by Mycobacterium tuberculosis. The lesions are produced and manifested by local proliferation to form tubercles and, by different diffuse exudation and proliferation processes which go under caseation, necrosis, ulceration or heal with fibrosis— calcification ensues thereafter.

This disease has been in existence since the early civilization of humanity. Indian ancient texts give a full account of this type of symptoms and they promise a complete cure of this disease. Ayurveda therapy has been there to treat this disease. "Yakshma" or "Rajyakṣhma" has been the identifying name of this dreadful disease.

Simultaneous to us Greek physicians made different observations on tuberculosis (specially pulmonary tuberculosis) right from the days of Hippocrates (460-377B.C.). Galen (130-210 A.D.), the great physician, diagnosed its infectious nature. F. Sylvius (1614-1672) hinted a close connection between tuberculous nodule and phthisis in seventeenth century. Franciscus investigated the pathogenic lesion made by the tubercle bacillus and named it "Tubercle". In modern age, Richard Morton is considered to be the first author who has aspected tuberculosis in its complete clinical sight. The important thing he noted — it is a contagious disease. Pierre Desault, William Stark and Mathew Baillie laid the anatomical basis of tuberculosis. They observed the deformities in human body due to this disease.

Franciscus's work was very important from the point of view of nomenclature of this disease, and later on Gaspard Lavrent Bayle named the disease "Tuberculosis". In nineetenth century, Bayle worked on the structure of tubercle also. In 1819, Laennec (1781-1826) laid the foundation of clinical characteristics of tuberculosis and its modern treatment. The physical sign of disease and course of the treatment find a systematic record in work of Laennec. It is an unfortunate but interesting fact that Laennec died of the disease - tuberculosis - he described so brilliantly in his book 'On Mediate Auscultation' (1819).

Villemin (1827-1892), experimentally showed the infectious nature of this disease. His work is considered to be more masterly in experimental medicine on this disease.

Finally, in 1882, Robert Koch (1843-1910) discovered the tubercle bacillus and proved that it was the cause of the disease known as tuberculosis. This was a great pathological finding and the years have gone but the scientific research of Robert Koch has stood unparallel.

Homoeopathically, if we think over the matter, we will find that in nineetenth century, our master Dr. Samuel Hahnemann (1755-1843) had discovered the cause of all chronic and long lasting diseases in concept of "MIASMS". The external bacillus may be the factor for sensitising tubercular pattern of symptoms in human body but it is not the final cause, (though it has a great potentiality. The finality lies in the germinating human body (soil), which allows the external seed to grow in it. This conclusion was more thought provoking, and now, after 200 years, at the dawn of twenty-first century, Dr. Hahnemann's approach to this infectious disease is more convincing and scientific. The reason is very simple. There are millions of microbes around us. They, certainly, happen to be infectious in so many cases. They are highly toxic and damaging, but to the point of wonder, we see, that some persons are infected and some not subject to condition that both classes of these persons were living in the same milieu. A child gets infection of tuberculosis through the sputum of his grandfather (who is tubercular) but, at the same time, the brother of that child, who lives in the same family and milieu, does not got infected. Why?

This is the efficacy of "Theory of Miasms" of homoeopathy. One person's body may be susceptible and vulnerable to Mycobacterium tuberculosis but not other's. The invading factor is the particular bacillus but it is the miasmatic state of homoeopathic philosophy which may or may not allow the growth and development of this particular microbe resulting in tuberculosis.

Many scientific discourses have taken place for knowing the real cause and nature of "MIASM", some has opined that it is a microbial interpretation of disease but some other has strongly opined that it is only one side of the coin, the other aspect of mysterious diathesis, which becomes sensitive to some external germ must never be lost sight of. The dyscrasia to catch and develop the symptoms is the real meaning of "miasms", is the latter's opinion.

Contemporary homoeopathic physicians and academicians take it granted that without dual interpretation of concept of "miasm" in cases of tuberuclosis, one cannot find the required success. In author's opinion the balanced view regarding both the aspects of "miasms" is much convincing and practical. The treatment of "tuberculosis" should be undertaken on this background.

Prevention (so that external factor may be kept away) and treatment (If there are predispositions to tubercular diathesis) are the balanced views to treat tubercular cases in homoeopathy.

2 The Accepted Premises of Tuberculosis in Homoeopathy

Before we look at the details of tuberculosis, some accepted premises of this disease will be aspected. These principles are commonly accepted by all homoeopathic physicians. It is true that the subtle sight and grasp of these principles will ensure the homoeopathic treatment of tuberculosis, successful.

1. The disease is caused by the organism Mycobacterium tuberculosis. This is the external factor.

2. The factor of "miasm" (Tubercular miasm) will have to be taken into consideration, whenever a case is to be treated by homoeopathic guidelines.

3. This external organism is killed by heat, sunlight and certain chemicals.

4. The sputum, saliva and the milk of animals suffering from tuberculosis have mostly organisms, of tuberculosis. They are the reservoirs of infection.

5. There is an inherent immunity against tuberculosis in each individual. Miasmatic sensitization completes the history and full cycle of this immunity.

6. Infants and youngs are more susceptible to tubercular infection.

7. Morbidity rates are high in the older age group of males.

8. Socio-economic status and nutrition play a major role in exciting the cause of tubercular diathesis.

9. The external contact and spread of infection is highly interlinked.

10. More the contact, more the possibility of infection.

11. An updated education regarding spread of tubercular infection and tuberculosis is a must, because it can prevent the further course of tuberculosis in other healthy or sensitized patients.

12. As has been written in older records that "tuberculosis is captain of death", so one should always keep in mind that no age is exempt in tuberculosis.

13. Radiological, haematological and dermal reactivity examinations are carried out to detect the disease. But we should always keep in mind that sometimes radiological examinations and dermal reactivities lack the susceptibility of tuberculosis.

14. A balanced observation of radiology, laboratory investigation, tuberculine testing, family history and mental-physical symptoms give an approach to detect the case of tuberculosis.

15. Poverty-pollution-low economic and living status with unhygienic sense, nexus form the breeding pool for tubercular cases.

16. Some races offer resistance to tuberculosis. This resistance varies from race to race and even from region to region. Africans, Indians, inhabitants of Western Isles of Scotland and of Ireland are more susceptible to tuberculosis.

17. It is by far the largest single cause of death in developing countries. About 66% deaths in India are due to tuberculosis.

18. From the word "tuberculosis" the sense is generally understood to that of pulmonary tuberculosis, but, in actuality, there are distinct other forms of tuberculosis in different organs of the human body.

19. Overcrowding is a very negative factor. Overpopulated inhabitations cause the most potent reason for spread of tubercular infection.

20. Dietary deficiencies of protein and vitamins are important aetiological factors of tuberculosis under certain other conditions.

21. Occupation has no direct bearing regarding tuberculosis except that the professionals of mining (as pneumoconiosis is there) and nursing (as heavy and massive infection is there) may develop in tubercular subjects.

22. Stress and strain for a tubercular patient are heavily unfavourable. These mental bearings deteriorate the case, hence tubercular patient should invariably lead a spiritual life.

23. If there are some other terminating and chronic disease already present in patient of tuberculosis, the management of the case, in that condition, requires a holistic approach and constitutional treatment. We should never forget that maintenance therapy is must in such type of cases.

24. A continuous respiratory irritation is a predisposition to tuberculosis pulmonali.

25. Previously it was a fatal disease and prognosis was very unfavourable, but, now-a-days, under medical supervision and proper treatment, it is fully controllable and treatable. Homoeopathic treatment of tuberculosis in early days or in beginning of the case is very successful. So as soon as the symptoms persist, homoeopathic techniques must be deployed to prevent any further complication.

26. If the vital principle is strong enough, in that condition, beside modern allopathic treatment, homoeopathic treatment can go side-by-side. Homoeopathy is competent enough to deal with the cases of tuberculosis.

27. "Prevention is better than Cure", is always a golden role in treatment or management of cases of tuberculosis.

28. About 50 years ago, this disease was the "Captain of death". This was a dangerous fatal disease, but now, the holistic approach to control, cure and treating this disease has made prognosis very favourable. Modern chemotherapeutic agents, laboratory investigation and mass propaganda have made it more controllable and curable. Homoeopathic drugs have also made a stride in this area. We have so many illustrations where a cure has been brought about by homoeopathic medicines.

There are five types of tubercle bacillus responsible for the disease, in man there are only two, but, again, we should keep in mind that these agents are external factors; if host has not a sending and germinating soil, they cannot grow.

Bacillis responsible as an external factor, responsible for the tuberculosis in man are

(a) The human type

(b) The bovine type

The human strain is responsible for vast majority of cases. As we know that Mycobacterium tuberculosis is a facultative intercellular parasite and as it is readily ingested by phagocytes and is resistant to intracellular killing; it is only the homoeopathic drugs action which can inhibit the tendency of the Mycobacterium. Fortunately, regarding virulence, Indian tubercle bacillus is less dangerous than the European bacillus.

Various researches have been conducted on tuberculosis, some other more important points have come in light :

1. Elderly males, generally between the age group 45-55, are more susceptible to

tuberculosis. Children below three years should be examined from the point of view of infection.

2. Females in higher age groups are generally not so susceptible, but below 35 years of the age there is a high risk factor.

3. It has been found more in low city-areas, slum-dwellers and lower socio-economic groups or families.

4. Tuberculine testing is widely used for estimating the prevalence of tuberculous infections.

5. Direct smear examination is considered a most relevant index for prevalance of tuberculosis of pulmonary site.

6. It is transmitted mainly by droplet infections. Coughing generates the largest number of droplets. It is not transmitted by fomites (substances capable of carrying infection), such as dishes and other articles used by the patient, latest researches have concluded. Unpasteurised milk is also potent cause for spread of bovine infection.

7. Patient with extrapulmonary tuberculosis or smear negative tuberculosis constitute a minimal hazard for transmission of infection.

8. Pre-Incubation period of infection in a tubercular diathesis case is generally from 3 to 6 weeks, and thereafter the development of tuberculosis depends upon the closeness of contact, extent of the disease and sputum positivity of the source case and host-parasite relationship. Thus incubation period may be weeks, months or years. This incubation, or the reception of infection by host, depends upon the miasmatic trend of patient. If the subject is not having tubercular diathesis, the disease may not get developed.

9. Tuberculosis affects all ages therefore be observant and careful to every open or susceptible case.

10. Elderly persons are more susceptible to tuberculosis in poor or developing countries.

11. Males are generally more affected than famales.

12. Though it is not a hereditary disease yet inherited susceptibility is an important risk factor. The concept of tubercular miasm and tuberculous diathesis provide some very helping instrument to assess the risk factor. The contribution of homoeopathy, in this field is great.

13. Malnutrition may have a potent effect if the invasion of Mycobacterium Tuberculosis has a more potent virulence factor.

14. Not undue exhaustion, fresh air, nutrition and good inhabitation are contributing positively to manage any case of tuberclosis.

15. Poor quality of life, poor housing, large families, early marriages, overcrowding, under-nutrition, lack of awareness and lack of education, all these factors are interrelated and contributing to tuberculosis. This is the reason why developing countries have by far the highest problems due to this disease.

16. Modern practice for prevention of tuberculosis is BCG Vaccination (Bacille Calmette - Guerin Vaccination). It is a safe preventive measure. In this, the living bacteria derived from an attenuated bovine strain of tubercle bacilli is introduced in optimum quantity. It is administered intradermally using a "tuberculin syringe". In India where childhood infection of tuberculosis is very high, it is introduced in infancy either at birth or at 6 weeks of age simultaneously with other immunizing agent such at DPT and polio. BCG administered early in infancy provides a higher level of proctection from

childhood tuberculosis and tuberculous meningitis. Sometimes at the site of BCG vaccination, ulceration and suppuration occurs, for this, vaccination should be strictly intradermal and for six month no injections should be given into that arm. The duration of protection of this BCG Vaccination is from 15 to 20 years. Whether booster dose is required or not is a matter of dispute, however, at school age, if booster dose be administered, it will protect from adult pattern tuberculosis. This type of vaccination has no side-effect even in tuberculine-positive reactors, according to W.H.O report. This is not a complete protection from tuberculosis, it can have only a relatively small epidemiological effect.

Though a consensus is yet to be reached in medical science but if homoeopathic drugs and nosodes be given right from pregnancy state to infancy, the child will be having a more thorough and long-lasting immunity from tuberculosis. Tuberculinum or Bacillinum, which are powerful nosodes, may prove a safe homoeopathic vaccine, if given from infancy stage to school age. Even if mother is given the protective doses of these nosodes at suitable intervals, her baby may be quite free from susceptibilities of childhood tuberculosis.

Psorinum, Syphilinum, Tuberculinum Medorrhinum and Schirinnum (Careinocin) are the major nosodes which may be given to mother at physician's advice to protect her baby from further complications. In this point, homoeopathists and physicians, different governments, gynaecologists and obstetricians must work. All these nosodes can save forthcoming generations from other ailments alongwith tuberculosis.

3 Common Indications for Tuberculosis and its Anatomical Sites

Homoeopathy treats the patient, not the disease; this is an unanimous accepted dictum of science of homoeopathy. The symptoms (physicals or pathophysicals) which are shown in tuberculosis are treated by homoeopathy. A peculiar symptom pattern of vital force may be tuberculosis or any other disease, but, in homoeopathy, if the same or similar symptom pattern exists in any disease (whatever be the name of disease), the same homoeopathic medicine works in different diseases very successfully.

Homoeopathy deals with the manifested symptomatology. The common indications in syndrome of tuberculosis are as under. A thorough understanding of all these points will reveal a good success :

1. Emaciation
2. Weight loss
3. Destruction of organ or system
4. Loss of appetite
5. Anaemia, debility
6. Malaise
7. Nightly sweats
8. Tachycardia
9. Pyrexia in afternoon or evening
10. Sub-febrile state

From local tubercular lesion, the tuberculosis of other anatomical organs may be developed. The majority of non-pulmonary tubercular lesions, other than lesions of the lymphatic glands, are haematogenous in origin. Local effects of the tuberculous lesions develop in different style on anatomical sites.

Anatomical Sites	**Physical Symptoms**
Lungs and Bronchi	Sputum, Cough, Haemoptysis, Dyspnoea
Pleura	Pain, Pleural effusion, Chest (Pleuritic pain) pain, Dyspnea due to pleural effusion
Larynx	Hoarseness, Dysphagia
Tongue, lips, tonsils	Ulceration
Intestines	Diarrhoea, Malabsorption, Intestinal obstruction
Peritoneum	Ascites, Intestinal obstructions
Pericardium	Pericardial effusion

Kidney and bladder	Haematuria, Increase urinary trend, Renal lesions occur erarly, later frequent micturition occurs
Epididymis	Painless swelling formation of sinus
Brain	Tuberculoma
Meninges	Meningitis pattern of symptoms
Suprarenal glands	Symptom pattern of Addison's disease
Bones and joints	Ostetitis, Synovitis, 'Cold' abscesses
Skin	Lupus vulgaris, Erythema nodosom
Eye	Phlyctenular kerato conjunctivitis, choroidits, Iridocycitis
Lymph nodes	Enlargement of Nodes, 'Cold abscesses' and formation of Sinus later on

In tuberculosis of these organs all the above referred symptoms are manifested accordingly.

Some other sites where tuberculosis may be developed are :
Complication of pulmonary tuberculosis in different organs.
Tuberculosis of Alimentary tract
Tuberculosis of Genito - urinary tract
Tuberculosis of Liver
Tuberculosis of Central Nervous system
Tuberculosis of Genital organ tract
Tuberculosis of Mammary glands
Tuberculosis of Circulatory system
Tuberculosis of Spleen
Tuberculosis of Heart
Tuberculosis of Endocrine glands (Thyroid, Pancreas and Hypophysis)

A detail of all these complications will be given at appropriate place. In particular organ's tuberculosis, the structural functional utility and working gets destructed and disturbed. The common symptoms of tuberculosis are manifested in different cases according to severity of disease.

Lungs, Pleura, Peritoneum, Pericardium, Meninges, Regional Lymph glands such as Cervical, Tracheobronchial and Mesenteric glands, Intestines, Larynx, Liver, Kidney, Spleen, Brain, Bone, Joints, Lips, Tongue, Palate, Tonsils, Fibrous tissues and Muscles,

Generalised tubercles usually known as acute Milliary tuberculosis are generally infected episodes of tuberculosis.

It should be kept in mind, though not be denied, that fibrous tissues and muscles get infected very rare by Mycobacterium Tuberculosis.

In adults, lungs are the common site of infection, whereas, in children, bones, joints and glands are usually affected. Tuberculosis of spine is also a comon site of infection in children.

4 Natural Course of Tuberculosis

Tuberculosis is an infectious disease. The genus Mycobacterium contains many organisms pathogenic to man and animals. The bacillus of tuberculosis is one of them in Mycobacterium genus.

Five typical varieties of M. tuberculosis extis, the human, the bovine, the piscine, the murine and the avian. The pathogens responsible for human infections are the human and bovine type. The avian is pathogenic for man only very rarely. The human type is found in pulmonary tuberculosis, where, as the bovine is found in tuberculosis of serous membranes, intestines, lymph nodes, bones and joints.

The human type is conveyed by inhaled droplets, where as the bovine by drinking infected milk. Sometimes skin abrasion also becomes a cause of spreading infection. It has been found that a dried sputum, which is away from sunlight, may have human type in it up to three years. Therefore contact with live case is responsible for this infection in human type. This is for pulmonary tuberculosis infection. Non-pulmonary infection occurs due to bovine type. Infection through suckling at breast has also been reported.

The theory of miasmatic susceptibility lies true in spreading and infecting the tuberculosis. The soil (as we find in some races or inhabitants of some regional area) resists, up to certain extent the infection. Numerous factors, as have been dealt with, previously, singly or in combination, act when man's resistance is overcome. Robust constitution, and vigorous general health are safeguards against tuberculosis. The natural resistance is lowered by unsanitary housing condition, lack of sunlight, exposure to weather and food deficiencies. The holistic approach of treatment of tuberculosis by homoeopathy has certainly got an unique role, when the factor of immunity is taken into consideration.

The important thing to be kept in mind is that organisms get into body through following modes :

1. Ingestion
2. Inhalation
3. Skin abrasion
4. Genito-urinary tract (sometimes)
5. Conjunctiva (rarely)

Therefore, precaution should be taken in these contacts.

It has also been found that no age is exempt for tuberculosis, however, puberty and pregnancy are physiological processes that seen to lower resistance.

It has also been observed and found correct that any debilitating disease, respiratory inflammation and continuous irritation lower the resistance and prepare the soil for further infection. The soil of diabetes mellitus is favourable to tubercle bacillus.

Alcoholism, Leukaemia, Arteriosclerosis, Cirrhosis of the liver and other diseases which are debilitating to body predispose to the development of tuberculosis. Pregnancy may also have an unfavourable influence on the course of untreated pulmonary tuberculosis.

Trauma as for example a blow on the chest, injury to knee, a blow upon the hand, may be followed by tuberculosis, as bacillus find a suitable ground for germination and development.

It has been repeatedly written that unhygienic condition of living and working contribute much for promotion of the disease.

Hereditary transmission of tuberculosis is under research, however, it has been found that tubercle bacilli can cross the placenta and cause tuberculosis of the fetus. Entry of the tubercle bacillus into the body may not be necessarily followed by clinical illness, but it depends on several other associating factors. It has, however, been proved that if a person contacts tuberculosis and recovers from primary imfection, he is less likely to develop active tuberculosis on subsequent exposure to bacillus than a patient who has not previously been infected. Man's natural resistance against tuberculosis is low in infancy, high in childhood, somewhat depressed in adolescence, and low again after forty, especially.

Primary infection recurs in early life, it may happen in the adult also. After the primary infection, the tissues react to the tubercle bacillus in a way that differs from their initial reactions. This is known as hypersensitivity to tuberculine. This is a complex process, but it localizes the infection at site, thus it acts as a strong defence. On the other hand, this allergic response due to power of producing caseation and liquefaction in the primary lesion and in the regional lymph nodes exerts an unfavourable influence on the course of the disease. Hypersensitivity may fade and disappear as lesions heal.

The physiological process of infection, immunity and allergy are very complex processes. In allopathic medicine there are so many beliefs regarding all these, but in homoeopathy the whole thing can be set right on the subtle understanding of miasmatic diathesis and concept of constitution. However, it should be kept in mind that a young child may receive tubercular infection from an open case of pulmonary tuberculosis, and it is the most susceptible age for infection, therefore all the precaution regarding same should be taken.

In all tubercles two processes go on,

The one is <u>Caseation</u> — destructive and dangerous

The other is, <u>Fibrosis</u> — conservative and healing

The ultimate result in any case depends upon which predominates. The characteristic lesion of tuberculosis is tubercle – a nodule, the specific lesion of tuberculosis. This consists of a microscopic nodular collection of epithelioid cells surrounded by zones of lymphocytes and fibroblasts. There may be giant cells and a few bacilli in the centre. Adjacent tubercles enlarge and coalesce at an early stage, this is followed by caseation—the destruction or necrosis. This lesion tends to heal by fibrosis and calcification. But, unfortunately, caseation and fibrosis process occur frequently.

The primary tuberculous infection occurs in lungs, or in tonsils or in alimentary tract specially in ileo-caecal region. These are accompanied by a caseous lesion in the regional lymph node. Sometimes, this primary infection fails to heal. This infection, during adoleseence or early adult life, may lead to a progressive pulmonary tuberculosis. When healing process is not complete, the tubercle bacilli come into blood stream, this phenomena develops the haematogenous lesions in lungs, bones, joints and kidneys. Such lesion develop after months or years of primary infection episode. When primary infection is not healed the infection may be carried by lymphatics from tuberculous mediastinal glands to pleura or pericardium. This produces pleurisy or pericarditis.

Sometimes the caseous tuberculous focus rupture into a vein and produces acute dissemination of the disease throughout the body. This is known as acute miliary tuberculosis. Tubercular meningitis often accompanies this condition. Extension of infection to pleura follows development of tuberculous emphysema, occasionally. Progressive pulmonary tuberculosis may get reactivation from an incompletely healed primary focus in the lung or as a result of haematogenous dissemination from an unhealed lymph node lesion. This is post-primary pulmonary tuberculosis or adult phthisis. In this tuberculous cavity is formed which contains numbers of tubercle bacilli. Fibrosis and calcification both the processes go slow. Extension of this infection reaches to other lung or different sites in the body.

The onset of generalised tuberculosis may be abrupt or gradual but initial symptoms are general. They are as :

Vague ill-health
Fatigue
Exhaustion
Headache
Weight loss (emaciation)
Fever

Anaemia in septicaemic form. When the disease establishes itself firmly the appearing physical symptoms are :

Fever (intermittent) 103°-104° F (40°C) in evening
Tachycardia
Pyrexia
Sweats at night
Insomnia
Headache
Profound prostration

After one to two weeks localising symptoms occur in two types; the "typhoid" and the "pulmonary". In the former, tumidity of abdomen occurrs. Liver and spleen become palpable, whereas, in the latter cyanotic flushes and dyspnoea. The possibilities of miliary tuberculosis and tubercular meningitis is not overruled. Pleural, or pericardial effusion, arthritis or cutaneous tuberculides may develop is succeesive crops over week or months and, finally, it may terminate into acute miliary tuberculosis and meningitis. In the septicaemic type toxaemia with progressive loss of weight, prostration and anaemia concludes the illness. Anthracinum, Pysogenium and Echinacea are the most important homoeopathic medicines for septicaemic stages.

The whole episode of "tuberculosis" and "infection" shows that the concept of "Constitution" and "Miasm" play a very important role. If the person's inhabitation is normal or sound, diet is normal, and if his diathesis is unfavourable to tubercular bacilli, he will never become a grave case. By homoeopathy, this possibility can be maintained.

5 The Diagnosis of Tuberculosis

The manifesting symptoms written earlier are a strong proof of tuberculosis in any person. Even if tuberculosis has not established and he is a negative case, even then, it is the tubercular diathesis, which may break out in tuberculosis in future.

So, for identifying the tubercular case, physical and patho-physical observations and laboratory investigations are done. If physical observation confirms the case, laboratory diagnosis must be carried out.

Laboratory diagnosis consists of two methods :

1. Direct Method
2. Indirect Method.

In direct method, tubercle bacillus test is carried out. The test materials are :

Sputum
Laryngeal swab
Pleural effusion
Gastric lavage
Faeces

In indirect method allergic reactions, tuberculin tests, and complement fixation test are carried out.

Direct Methods consist of :

1. Smear and Acid-fast staining of sputum
2. Culture
3. Animal inoculation (In guinea-pig)

Indirect methods consist of :

1. Blood picture – Lymphocytosis and Monocytosis
2. E. S. R. high
3. Tuberculin test
4. Complement fixation test

In Tuberculin test, the tuberculin–which is an extract from tubercle bacilli, and contains tuberculous protein and other material–is injected in small quantity. In a healthy person there is no reaction, hardly a negligible inflammation. occurs, but in an infected person it manifests oedema, erythema, induration and formation of pseudopodia at the site of injection. If it happens within 72 hours, it is a positive tuberculin reaction.

Mantoux test is a tuberculine test, which is carried out by intracutaneous method. The material which is injected contains old tuberculin (O. T.) or purified protein derivative (P. P. D.). But in Mantoux test OT is used. This is a test which is generally held out but sometimes it gives positive result with ageing whilst the person has no infection. In the earlier stages of disease, it may be negative. Only in very acute or advanced cases are the positive tests found. Some tuberculine tests are :

1. Mantoux test (Intradermal test) as explained earlier
2. Live test
3. Multiple puncture
4. Subcutaneous
5. Patches of jelly method
6. Cutaneous scarification
7. Ophthalmic

Complete fixation test with WKK antigen shows positive result in pulmonary tuberculosis, but it is true up to 70-80% in cases and that too in chronic cases.

REMEMBER, IT IS MOST IMPORTANT, THAT

If tuberculin test is positive, it means

1. Active disease
2. 4-6 week past infection
3. In a serial study, if it has converted from negative to positive it means active disease
4. Potentiality of host to develop the disease.

Sometimes, due to presence of other mycobacteria, it may be positive, but it is false. In children below three years, if it comes positive, it means active disease in the patient.

If tuberculin test is negative, it means

1. There is no contact with tubercle bacillus.
2. As individual has got no immunity to the disease, so he is more susceptible to disease
3. Negativity of the test should be confirmed from continuous six week's test, even on using higher concentration of tuberculin material.

Tuberculin tests are important for confirming the situation, early diagnosis, specially in children, screening and efficacy test for BCG administration and mass surveillance.

When we talk about mass surveillance, the case finding tests (tools) are :

1. Sputum examination
2. Mass miniature radiography
3. Tuberculin tests

Radiological findings (X-rays) are always not true, so the lesions of X-rays should be confirmed with some other means.

In cases of tuberculosis of bones (which is most common in India) besides the referred tests, some other laboratory tests are : Biopsy of regional lymph node and Exploratory arthrotomy—which is the certain way of examining the disease, Radiographic test, CT Scan and MRI.

These all are laboratory techniques to confirm the disease on physical plane. A homoeopathist may get help from these tests. But as we know that a true homoeopathist should command the clinical methods so a subtle sight on patho-physiological symptoms and then, if they are positive, an administration of "similimum" is the most powerful tool in hands of any homoeopathist. Beside the external techniques, a homoeopathist's view and his confirmation of tubercular miasm will undoubtedly open the case, it is beyond any doubt.

6 Respiratory Tuberculosis

Respiratory tuberculosis is related with pulmonary tuberculosis. It is most frequently observed in daily practice. It has been indicated that respiratory tuberculosis is the action result of mycobacterium tuberculosis.

It is an infectious and inflammatory disease caused by the tubercle bacillus, where formation of tubercle, abscess, cavities, necrotic caseation, fibrosis and calcification occur. This is the infection which may be caused by way of droplet inhalation or gastrointestinal tract.

A close contact with an open case of tuberculosis where the sputum of that patient is projected into air, and invisible thousands of microorganism of tuberculosis are inhaled by swallowing that sputum. Children generally catch infection in their families in this manner. By drinking infectious milk, the infection may also develop.

The common indication and course of the disease have already been described earlier.

PRIMARY PULMONARY TUBERCULOSIS

Primary infection occurs mostly in children or in early life but adults are also not immune to same.

In primary days, no symptoms are manifested; later on, in some cases, a slight fever devclops for 7 to 14 days and a slight dry cough is present. If the subject is suffering from any infectious disease like typhoid fever or illness like whooping cough, pleurisy, pneumonia, or any eruptive fever, the susceptibility to catch infection increases as these disease lower the resistance. Moreover, if inhabitation (milieu) is unhygienic and downgraded and food is not properly nutritious, the susceptibility to catch infection is more. Too frequent pregnancies and too long continued nursing may also be a factor instigating susceptibility.

The primary focus is not always in respiratory system. It may be in abdomen, middle ear, genital organs or superficially on the skin or conjunctivae. Primary focus of these sites may also be in intestinal mucous membranes, abdominal lymph nodes, tonsils or cervical lymph nodes. This is primary complex phenomenon.

THE LEADING SYMPTOMS OF THIS STATE ARE

1. Pyrexia, malaise, headache,
2. Chest symptoms—cough, pain
3. Abdominal disturbances
4. Appearance on skin the eruptions—the erythema nodosum
5. Pleural effusion

These primary signs may be dormant for months or weeks, but later on they manifest. E. S. R is always high in blood test. Tuberculin test is positive. Skin eruption may be in other similar diseases also, so blood examination and radiological examination must confirm tuberculosis. In some cases, this primary complex process goes unnoticed and heals automatically but, later on, it may extend and cause extensive destruction and cavitation.

Mostly the primary infection in the lung may be bronchogenic, hematogenous or lymphatic route or combination of these. This entry may be mostly by inhalation.

Unfavourable signs of this infection are emaciation, persistent high rate of E.S.R, prolonged pyrexia, persistent tachycardia. If they or other complications such as Erythema nodosum (skin eruption), pleurisy (dry or with effusion), bronchiectasis, swollen gland and visceration of the same and, later on, the infection leads to miliary tubercle and tuberculous meningitis or tubercular disease in other organs for example the skeletal genito-urinary tract, kidney, liver and spleen.

Common indications shown in previous chapters are generally found in primary infection. A homoeopath is competent enough to observe those and treat accordingly. Radiological examination, Tuberculin test, Blood investigations, Bacteriological examination and Sputum examination show the pathological positivity of tuberculosis. Haemoptysis and breathlessness also develop as the disease increases. In early stages, there may not be morning temperature, but, in advanced cases, morning temperature may be higher or a pattern of remittent or intermittent fever may exist. It has been said earlier, that miliary tuberculosis and tubercular meningitis may complicate the picture at any stage.

It should also be kept in mind that in young adults the virulence of primary infection is more severe. A recent infection in young adult reinfects the system it is more severe. There is a blending of exudative and productive lesions in this type. Caseation and cavitation occur, fibrosis occurs but calcification is too less in such type (reinfected cases).

MILIARY TUBERCULOSIS

It occurs mainly in children and young adults. The tubercle lesions spread in whole of the body. It shows a similar onset with relative bradycardia and palpable spleen. It may be preceded by a few weeks of vague ill health.

The leading symptoms are :

1. Pyrexia (recurrent)
2. Drenching sweats during sleep
3. Tachycardia
4. Cough, Dyspnoea, Anorexia
5. Marked anaemia, loss of weight
6. Pleuritic pain
7. Enlarged glands (sometimes)

The above symptoms show a tubercular situation. Laboratory test of blood anaemia, leucocytosis and tuberculin test of sputum and stool and radiological examination confirm the activity of disease. In this situation tuberculosis of progressive nature in pulmonary region may develop. The formation of tubercle foci, then caseation, then abscess formation are found in miliary tuberculosis. The formation of cavities decides the progressive pulmonary tuberculosis. They are commonly situated in the upper lobes.

POST-PRIMARY PULMONARY TUBERCULOSIS

It has been said earlier, progressive pulmonary tuberculosis has lesions most commonly in upper lobes and at the apex of a lower lobe. The disease starts from one lung and spreads to the other.

The onset of the disease is usually insidious; the common indication of tuberculosis appear in the case. Cough, sputum or sudden haemoptysis, pleurisy or a spontaneous pneumothorax heralds the onset of the disease.

THE LEADING SYMPTOMS OF THE DISEASE ARE

1. Cough—sometimes unexplained
2. Sputum
3. Haemoptysis
4. Dyspnoea on exertion
5. Pleurtic pain
6. Pleursy with or without effussion
7. On examining lung consolidation, cavitation and fibrosis may appear; unexplained tiredness, loss of weight.

It has also been found that unexplained cough, loss of weight, tiredness without any respiratory problem, haemoptysis and chest pain should be suspected with the existence of disease.

For homoeopathy, these symptoms are quite sufficient to prescribe a suitable medicine. However, radiological examination, bacteriological examination of sputum and laboratory examination may confirm the pathological state of the disease.

If the case is left untreated some complications may appear, they may be as under:

- Depression
- Malaise—undue fatigue.
- Fever
- Toxaemia
- Rise of temperature, generally after afternoon
- Chilliness
- Denching night sweats
- Increased pulse
- Systolic B. P. lowers diastolic B. P. remains generally stable
- Flushing of the face
- Increased respiration
- Cyanosis
- Constipation and diarrhoea, diarrhoea is usually observed in advanced case
- Menstruation altered—Amenorrhea
- Libido and potentia remain stable

- Emaciation, Loss of weight
- Sharp cutting chest pain
- Cough is, as usual, a common symptom
- Dyspnoea
- Haemoptysis—sputum may have blood
- Husky vioce
- Greyish, catarrhal mucus
- Sudden haemoptysis
- The affeted side shoulder and breast, nipple are lower in strata. Asymmetry of scapula, Curvature in spine, Trapezius (muscular) atrophy; Atrophy of the shoulder girdle muscle of affected side. Pleurisy with or without effusion, chest expansion reduced.

The complications of pulmonary disease, may it be of any of the above type, or, in post-primary pulmonary tuberculosis, may manifest the symptoms but, meanwhile, it should also be kept in mind that

- Diabetics develop tuberculosis (pulmonary)
- Hyperthyroidism is bad for pulmonary tuberculosis
- Pulmonary tuberculosis should be avoided and, if pregnancy is there, every care must be taken, better if one waits for inactivity of tubercular lesions for two years.
- Pneumonia may develop
- Typhoid fever may develop
- Eruptive fevers, measles etc. may develop
- Fistula-in-ano develop
- Apart from the bacillus (phthisis) some other microorganism like streptococci and pneumococci develop to complicate degenerate and inflame the situation.
- Toxaemia develops
- Cardiovascular disease and all forms of congenital heart diseases may develop pulmonary tuberculosis
- Chronic renal disease
- Repeated haemoptysis is very unfavourable
- Erythema nodosum develops

Therefore, every precaution should be taken for curing and controlling the disease. If patient is not given a proper treatment he may die out of :

Haemorrhage
Coma-Cerebral thrombosis
Asthenia
Syncope
Asphyxia.

Therefore every prophylaxis measure should be taken. Some of the following or some similar complication in advanced pulmonary tuberculosis may be developed, they should also be kept in sight

1. Depression.

2. Pigmentation or eruption on skin.
3. Anaemia and Diarrhoea, Anorexia.
4. Destruction of extensive areas of lungs—gangrene of the lung.
5. Exertional dyspnoea.
6. Ventilatory failure.
7. Pulmonary heart disease.
8. Chronic ill-health due to secondary infection by pyogenic bacteria of damaged lung tissue
9. Tuberculous enteritis may develop after swallowing infected sputum
10. Tuberculous laryngitis may develop due to constant contact of bacilli loaded cough. Deglutition difficult
11. Ischio-rectal abscess and fistula in ano may develop due to constant passing of bacilli loaded material through the abrasion in the rectal mucosa
12. Tuberculous pus formation, and suppurative pneumonia may develop; ear may also be infected.
13. Dissemination of tuberculosis through the blood stream may cause renal tuberculosis or tuberculosis meningitis.
14. Amenorrhea; Hypertrophy of mammary gland.

These complications are organic and pathological in character. They may be well-controlled by giving organotherapic doses. Some bronchial and pulmonary disease, or some neoplasms (growth) or some mycotic infection and abscess formation should not be misdiagnosed as pulmonary tuberculosis. However, if it is misdiagnosed, the homoeopathic medicine selected for tuberculosis will work for these misdiagnosed conditions also, provided it be a similimum to manifesting symptoms.

It has been mentioned that the best way to treat tuberculosis is as soon as the symptoms are manifested, the constitutional homoeopathic medicine and one of the selected tuberculosis medicine should be started. It can prevent further losses.

Arsenic, Cal-carb, Bryonia, Tuberculinum, Dulcamara, Kali-carb, Hycopodium, Stannum, Silica, Sanguinaria, Nit-ac, Ars-iod, Apis, Apocyn, Iodoform, Zincum, Acalypha and Yerba santa are commonly used homoeopathic remedies for all the above complications and diseases.

7 Non-Respiratory Tuberculosis

Non-respiratory tuberculosis contains all those organs' affection with tuberculosis which do not take part directly in respiratory process.

Non-respiratory tuberculosis are generally haematogenous in nature. These patients may have tuberculosis somewhere else in their body and, later on, by stimulating or due to secondary infection, tuberculosis in other organs is manifested. However, it is not always a rule, primary infection may also be there, even direct invasion of bacillus may be there.

Common indication of tuberculosis and symptoms of tuberculosis are generally and clearly mixed with the organic dysfunctional symptoms. Constitutional tuberculosis treatment is must in these cases with other ancillary management.

Following is a list and brief description of non-respiratory tuberculosis.

TUBERCULOSIS OF LYMPH NODES

Scrofola is the other name for this type of tubercular infection to lymph nodes. However it is not a proper word. In this tuberculosis, different glands are involved.

The lymph node of the lymphatic drainage system form a focus of tuberculosis. The lymph nodes of neck, at the bifurcation of bronchi or those of the mesentery may be involved.

Healing occurs finally through a long battle between pathological development–enlargement of nodes and defense goes on before. Suppuration occurs after sinus formation or ulceration.

Fever, malaise, anorexia and other common symptoms of tuberculosis may be there. It has been found that lymphatic, lymph and lymphoid tissue are the defence soldiers of the body. The reticuloendothelial system has a great closeness with lymph system.

Homoeopathic concept of vital force can be understood in terms of joint venture of RES (Reticuloendothelial system) and PsNES (Psycho Neuro Endocrine system). Whenever there is invasion of tubercle bacilli in human body a close association between lymph nodes and system and reticuloendothelial system has been seen.

Whenever the tubercle bacillus invades blood stream and reach lymphs they form a lymph node focus. In this action lungs, spleen, kidneys, liver and serous membranes get affected. In time lymph nodes, particularly auircular, cervical, axillary, epitrochlelar inguinal and mediastinal enlarge and the spleen becomes palpable. Serous effusion (Bryonia) appears in pleura or peritoneum. Genitourinary tuberculosis may develop and often papulonecrotic tuberculides of the skin, multiple bone and joint lesions or eye lesions give a clue that the defence system of body is fighting with tuberculosis.

At this time fever of unknown origin, fatigue, malaise, and weight loss occur.

When the infiltration and deposition of tubercle bacillus become more concentrated, pathological and physiological changes take place; these latent symptoms go unnoticed for sometime, but the general symptoms of low fever and under-nourishment are seen.

Latently, tuberculosis goes on in this process scattering small foci and five nodules in different organs of the body. The process of subacute generalized lymphohaematogenous or its chronic and latent form goes in the body.

Any homoeopathist, when shown the physical symptoms of anaemia, fatigue, fever and malaise, prescribes the homoeo medicine, which starts work even for those sub-acute or latent stages which have not been diagnosed clearly.

TUBERCULOUS LYMPHADENITIS

The tuberculosis of gland is not very rare among tuberculosis patients. Mostly tuberculosis of glands is found in following glands :

Cervical
Tracheobronchial
Mesenteric

Tuberculous cervical adenitis is found among the children. Nodular eruption and lump enlargement of gland, inflammation and oedematous swelling, suppuration occurs. Coryza, eczema of the scalp ear or lips with conjuctivitis, keratitis are general symptoms. Fever may also be there.

The glands affected in this tuberculosis are of :

1. Sub-maxillary group (Near upper or lower Jaw-bone area)
2. Carotid group (Neck gland area)
3. Submeatal and submandibular group (Near chin and jaw-bone area)
4. Pre-auricular gland (Near ear area)
5. Groups of glands in the posterior and suprascapular region (Above the shoulder blade area)

THE LEADING SYMPTOMS ARE

1. Oedema
2. Swelling
3. Enlarged size
4. Often painless in beginning phase
5. Sinus or Ulcer formation
6. Pus secretion.

This infection may give rise to Tuberculosis of mammary glands in aged females. Continuous nasal catarrh, recurrent other infections are susceptible ground for the infection in children.

Tuberculous tracheobronchial adenitis is manifested by enlarged nodes, irregular fever, failure of nutrition, loss of appetite, lassitude, paroxysmal cough, fever, pain in mammary region.

Tuberculous mesenteric adenitis is manifested by enlargement of nodes of the mesentery and retroperitoneum. It is usually found in children. It may be a primary or secondary to tuberculosis of the intestines. In adults, it occurs with association of pulmonary tuberculosis or as a primary affection. The right side of umbilicus is felt with little tumor. The general symptoms are slight fever, local pain, sometimes diarrhoea and appendicitis is often suspected. But it is tough to diagnose it separately from other abdominal diseases. In this tuberculosis involvement of mesenteric gland occurs through primary infection of the intestines. The leading symptoms of this disorder are—

1. Vague ill health
2. Malaise
3. Abdominal pain in right iliac pssa
4. Nausea
5. Vomiting
6. Anorexia
7. Emaciation
8. Pyrexia of unknown origin
9. Anaemia
10. Constipation
11. Diarrhoea and abdominal pain.

Bovine type of bacilli may be found mostly in tuberculosis of lymph nodes, bones and joints; and human type in pulmonary affection. This categorization is based on the way and mode of spread of infection. From inhalation the virulent droplets and swallowing infected milk, human and bovine type reach human body, respectively.

TUBERCULOSIS OF ENDOCRINE GLANDS

The endocrine glands influence growth, metabolism reproduction and many bodily processes, especially with the involvement of central nervous system.

Tuberculosis of tuberculous destruction or atrophy is found in Adrenal, Thyroid Hypophysis and Pancreas.

In tuberculosis of ***hypophysis*** the disease pattern of Simond's disease (the endocrine disease pattern) whereas in tuberculosis of ***thyroid gland***, thyroiditis and enlargement of gland is seen. In tuberculosis of ***adrenal gland***—the Addison's disease pattern (anaemia, general langour, remarkable feebleness of heart's action, irritability of the stomach and a peculiar change of the colour in the skin, weight loss, nausea, vomiting, headache, confusion, severe pain in back or legs, subfebrile state, blood pressure falls to very low, urine diminishes and coma may be present in this tuberculosis).

Homoeopathic treatmant of tuberculosis of endocrine gland is wholly constitutional. The tubercular medicines which have been narrated later in this work are worth reliable according to symptoms. For endocrine treatment, readers are advised to go through the author's work "Understanding Gland, Endocrinology the Homoeopathic approach" published by B. Jain Publishers, New Delhi, for a better and uptodate care and cure. This tuberculosis requires constitutional treatment more than any other.

TUBERCULOSIS OF CENTRAL NERVOUS SYSTEM

Tubercular meningitis is due to the infection of the meninges from an infected caseous focus in the brain. Primary lesion of tuberculosis may be situated in bones, joints, lungs or gastrointestinal tract.

This is an infection of meninges with bacillus tuberculosis. Ischemia of brain tissues may occur.

The leading symptoms of tubercular meningitis are—

1. Headache–the predominant symptom
2. Restlessness nature
3. Apathetic
4. Loss of weight
5. Pyrexia of unknown origin
6. Drowsiness
7. Night meningeal cry
8. Vomiting
9. Strabismus–corneal opacity
10. Necrosis and degeneration of brain tissue occur in later stages
11. Hemiplegia or paraplegia.

Pathological check up of cerebral spinal fluid, bacteriological test of microbe and examination of blood (Monocytosis and High E.S.R.) diagnose the case of tuberculus meningitis.

In primary stages, headache is the key note symptom, but, later on, deterioration of brain tissue and paralysis occur. If acute headache is associating CSF test positive and finely seeded miliary disease in lungs, it is a confirmation of tubercular meningitis. That is why the above-referred tests are carried out.

For homoeopathy, the manifesting headache, restlessness, aphasia, and other neurological signs count much. The above-referred general symptoms point towards homoeopathic medicines. It will be seen that infection and degeneration are the chief symptoms. If tubercular meningitis is associated with miliary tuberculosis, the constitutional treatment is required.

Classical symptoms which are common to any form of tuberculosis should always be kept in mind for selecting the medicine.

TUBERCULOSIS OF THE LIVER

Liver is infected with infection in miliary tuberculosis.

The leading symptoms of this disease are :

1. Enlarged liver
2. Rough tender liver
3. Jaundice
4. Pus formation; abscess
5. Liver cirrhotic process.

In all the chronic forms of tubercule in this organ there may be fibrous overgrowth; common symptoms of tuberculosis may be accompanying this disorder.

TUBERCULOSIS OF THE SPLEEN

Chronic cases of splenomegaly (enlargement of spleen) with cyanosis and polycythemia are manifested in tuberculosis of spleen. It is a very rare affection. Tuberculosis pain in splenic region is also associated.

TUBERCULOSIS OF THE EYE

A pattern of symptoms as met in conjunctivitis is seen in tuberculosis of eye. Phyctenular conjunctivitis is seen. The disease usually commences in conjunctiva of the upper lid, occurs in young subject and only in one eye.

The following general symptoms are watched in disease.

1. Thickening of eyelids
2. Swelling, pain
3. Reddening of eye
4. Lachrymation
5. Photophobia
6. Nodular appearance in conjuctiva
7. Ulceration—necrosis.

This is primary infection. Perosteitis and caries of the orbit, tubercular nodule in the eyelids, conjunctiva, iris and choroid, tuberculous iridocylitis, iritis with greyish red nodules and phyctenular kerato conjunctivitis, all have been seen in tuberculosis of eyes. Several children suffering from skeletal tuberculosis have corneal opacities. This corneal opacity may be the result of tubercular conjunctivitis, with which the child has been loaded earlier. Tubercular choroiditis may be the result of miliary tuberculosis.

For homoeopathic treatment in this disease, the factor of tubercular miasm and syphilitic miasm must be considered.

TUBERCULOSIS OF ALIMENTARY TRACT

This tuberculosis accompaines tuberculosis elsewhere, especially in lungs.

Tuberculosis of lips has ulceration on lips with or without pulmonary tuberculosis. The cheeks, gum and floor of the mouth very rarely are involved. Lupus occasionally extends to the mouth from the skin.

Tuberculosis of tongue has ulceration, an irregular, rough caseous base sore. It is generally found with pulmonary tuberculosis.

Tuberculosis of salivary glands has inflammation and swelling and a chronic fibroid on parotid glands.

Tuberculosis of palate is manifested after neighbouring extension. The lesions are found which are multiple and ulcerated.

Tuberculosis of tonsils has superficial ulceration, pain, difficulty in swallowing. From this site, tuberculosis extends to cervical glands.

Tuberculosis of pharynx has ulceration. It is an extension of tuberculosis from the epiglottis, larynx or tonsils. Deglutition is painful. Adenoids of the nasopharynx may be tuberculous.

TUBERCULOSIS OF ESOPHAGUS :

Tuberculosis of stomach has prominent ulcers. Perforation may occur. Extra gastric lymph node lesions may extend into stomach. Miliary tuberculosis may be present.

Tuberculosis of abdomen is associated with tuberculous peritonitis of miliary origin, tuberculous salpingitis, tuberculous peritonitis, tuberculosis of the caecum, suprarenal tuberculosis, tuberculous appendicitis and tuberculosis of liver and spleen.

Tuberculous peritonitis is haematogenous in origin. It is closely associated with pleurisy or pleural effusion. Both may be present in same patient. The leading symptoms are ***fever, pain, abdominal restlessness*** and ***pain, vomiting, ascitic stage*** may be present. Diarrhoea may be present. Intestinal ulceration is not a characteristic feature of tuberculous peritonitis. Pulmonary tuberculosis may be associated with tubercular peritonitis.

Tuberculous salpingitis occurs between 20 and 40 in females. It is haematogenous in origin. It contains of the inflammation of fallopian tubes. From this site, tuberculosis may spread to peritoneum.

Tuberculosis of caecum occurs as an ulcerative process of the mucous membrane of the ileocaecal region or as a hyperplastic tuberculosis of the submucous and muscular wall of the caecum. The regional mesenteric glands become enlarged and may caseate. Associated tuberculous lesions in other parts of the body may be present.

The leading symptoms of tuberculosis of caecum are ***colic of small intestine, pain localized to the lower right quadrant of the abdomen, diarrhoea;*** in later stage, ***anorexia, low grade fever, loss of weight,*** hyperpigmentation of exposed skin surface, fistulae and clubbing of finger are found.

The similar situations may occur in appendicitis, appendix abscess, ileitis, carcinoma of the caecum, ulcerative colitis extending into ileum and caecal amoebiasis.

Homoeopathic treatment in any of the above situations selects the "similimum" as per the manifested symptoms. Some patients may have ***tubercular appendicitis*** associated with pulmonary tuberculosis in secondary infection. ***Tuberculosis of liver and spleen*** is also developed by haematogenous tubercular disease. There is also a possibility of ***tuberculosis of suprarenals*** where classical pigmentation of the skin on the exposed surfaces, cardiovascular asthenia and gastro-intestinal obstruction or disturbances are found.

The whole phenomena revolves around the symptom patterns for homoeopathists. There may be mistakes in diagnosis of particular ailments, and, thus, in treatment from allopathic point of view, but, for homoeopathy, there is no room for such type of misdiagnosis. A subtle grasp of characteristic symptom pattern opens the whole case. Cuprum-met, plumbum-met, Merc-sol, and intestinal Bach nosodes may be helpful in tuberculosis of intestines as a whole and, equally, in particular pathological deformity and dysfunctioning of lower gastro-intestinal tract.

TUBERCULOSIS OF THE KIDNEY

Renal tuberculosis is mostly haematogenous in origin and is a local manifestation of pre-existing neighbouring focus. It is an extension of miliary tuberculosis. Both the kidneys are affected.

In the male, renal tuberculosis infection spreads to urinary tract and from there it spreads to genital system. Infection of pelvis, bladder, epididymes, seminal vesicles and prostate are the sites. Females between 30-40 years of age are usually infected.

The leading symptoms of tuberculosis of kidney are :

1. Frequent micturition
2. Urgent and painful micturition
3. Albuminuria occurs, urine pale, turbid, traces of pus may be there, acidic in reaction.
4. Haematuria
5. Lumbar pain.

In infection of tuberculosis of this organ an external invasion is never found. It is also found that in other patients who have some other form of tuberculosis pass bacillus in their urine, but infection does not occur in renal area. The primary focus in the kidney is formed in the cortex related to glomeruli. From other sites it invades the renal area.

In male persons, infection is carried out from bladder to the male genital organs through the vehicle of urine : therefore it gets converted into tuberculosis of genito-urinary tract. In genital sphere, infection starts from prostate gland; later on seminal vesicles, epididymis, testes. In males, therefore, tuberculosis spreads from renal to the genital system.

The development of the renal lesion depends on the quanta of invading bacilli :

1. Any acute pyogenic urinary infection
2. Pain
3. Burning
4. Difficulty in micturition and later on frequency of micturition
5. Bleeding
6. Congestion, inflammation of bladder wall
7. Haemorrhage from kidney cause intense colic
8. Dull ache in loin
9. Pain in suprapubic and rectum
10. If the infection is limited to only genital tract, both testes become swollen
11. Malaise
12. Weight loss
13. Fatigue and depression
14. Pathological finding in urine—albumin, pus, red blood cells, acidic in reaction. If the quanta of pus increases, it is a sign of progress of the disease of tuberculosis pertaining to genito-urinary tract
15. If disease advances, renal functions are lost, the patient will complain of thirst and loss of appetite. Uraemia and smell in urine may also be there.

Here it must be noticed that common indications of tuberculosis may be present in tuberculosis of genito-urinary tract. Genital tuberculosis in the females is not particularly associated with renal disease but is a more common complication of phthisis than is generally recognized for the symptoms and signs are not usually conspicuous. In women, genital tuberculosis manifest inflammation, salpingo-oorphoritis and metritis; bladder symptoms may arise because of the close proximity of the affected organ.

Tuberculosis of ureter and bladder is primary but nearly always secondary to involvement of other parts, particularly the kidney. The renal regions, the testes, the seminal vesicles and the prostate should be examined with care. Stone formation may be there. Tuberculosis of Ureter always accompanies tuberculosis of the kidney.

Tuberculosis of prostate, vesiculae seminals and penis. The prostate may be nodulous, the seminal vesicles become thick, enlarged, tender and nodular.

Tuberculosis of testis and epididymis is a network of tuberculosis of adjacent organs. Trauma and previous inflammation may be the disposing factor. Painless enlargement is found; later on pain occurs, sexual desire remains unchanged, azo-spermia is frequent. Semen may contain tubercle bacilli.

Nodular growth, pain and inflammation occur in all these tuberculosis.

So far as the female organs are concerned ***tuberculosis of fallopian tubes, ovaries and uterus*** needs a great concern. Salpingitis (inflammation of fallopian tube). Ulceration, formation of abscess occurs. Tuberculosis of uterus is rare but if it occurs it is associated with tuberculosis of lungs. Vagina may also be affected; with pulmonary tuberculosis, placenta is affected.

Tuberculosis of Mammary gland occurs between fortieth and sixtieth years of age. The fistulae and ulcer may be there as manifestation of tuberculosis.

For homoeopathic symptomatology it is said that along with general symptomatology of tuberculosis, renal pain, frequency of urination, bleeding, unpleasant smell in urine and turbidity of urine point out to homoeopathic medicine. On this symptoms, the real medicine can be searched out. If genital tract is involved sexual dysfunctionalism in both the sexes is easy to watch and act upon homoeopatically.

It should also be kept in mind that infection of genito-urinary tract may be congenital, therefore, if mother is infected, or positive, the children also should be treated.

TUBERCULOSIS OF SKIN

Tuberculosis of skin is a direct result of infection (primary or secondary). The skin manifests various growths of lesions.

Tubercular patients who have miliary tuberculosis or tuberculous lesions of the lung, or other organs and tissues may develope skin symptoms, therefore while examining any case of tuberculosis one should be quite vigilant.

The general symptomatology of these eruptions are

1. Lesions
2. Sometimes dry
3. Erythema
4. Pus secretion

5. Reddened in colour
6. Necrotic character
7. Ulceration
8. Scar formation
9. Hyperpigmentation.

These problems can be very well reportorized in homoeopathy. The tubercular eruptions which have been described below have the general symptomatology, as written above.

Homoeopathy has got a very special say in dermatological problems. The occurrence of their site is additionally helpful for homoeopathists, as homoeopathy has those type of medicines which have special anatomical site modality.

A better way to treat them is the constitutional treatment and also caring of the dermal disorders. Local treatment should never be encouraged as it may aggravate the tubercular process.

The external agent Mycobacterium tuberculosis is implanted directly on the skin through gastro-intestinal tract, respiratory system or abrasion of skin. If the subject is having any susceptibility to tuberculosis dyscrasia, the infection is established.

Tuberculosis of skin is manifested in following manner—

1. When the subject has not been primarily exposed to bacillus and has no hypersensitivity to tuberculin, the nondescriptive brownish painless nodule breaks down within seven or eight days of contact. This occurs when bacillus implants into the skin directly. It is found on open parts of body. Regional lymph nodes are enlarged; finally a ragged ulcer with undermined edges and haemorrhage occur. This is known as ***tubercular chancre.***
2. Where a high degree of inmunity to bacillus is there, ***Lupus Vulgaris*** the most common eruption occurs. The face is the most common place where it occurs. It is like an apple-jelly nodule. Primarily it manifests as multiple erythematous, irregular in durated plaque(s). Ulceration and scar formation may occur. These lesions slowly extend irregularly at the periphery. The lesion, occasionally, is more verrucous and dry and comprises of large number of soft nodules. Buttocks, groins, shoulders, trunk and glans penis are other sites for these lesions face, lupus vulgaris, if left standing for a long time, may develop carcinoma. The physical expression of these eruptions is like small, dull red, pinhead size spot, surrounded by a zone of erythema finally, ulceration may develop from these soft jelly like nodules.

   Alike lupus vulgaris, eruptions which are more verrucous are called ***tuberculosis verrucosa cutis.*** It has erythema around its eruption. This distinguishes it from the general wart. It is usually found on the dorsum of the hand or feet.
3. ***Scrofuloderma*** occurs on the skin where in lymph glands, bones or joints lies tubercular infection. The skin becomes swollen and reddened. The lesions developed thereafter consist of single or multiple sinuses with undermined edges which discharge thin yellow pus. These are, sometimes, surrounded by lupus vulgaris. Scarring of lesion produces irregular mass. Pus is discharged.

The site of these lesions are near lymph nodes bones or joints.

4. ***Lichenscrofulosorum*** develops through haematogenous way. They develop from other infectious sites. Small coloured papules occur on skin. They heal after a long time without scarring. Trunk of children is the common site for their occurrance.
5. ***Orificial tuberculosis*** occurs due to direct inoculation of bacillus of tuberculosis on oral, anal or urogenital mucosae of the patients suffering from tuberculosis of lungs, gastro-intestinal tract or kidney. Multiple painful shallow ulcers with undermined edges are present in this affection. These are found in very advanced cases of tuberculosis.
6. ***Papulo-Necrotic tuberculosis.*** It spreads through haematogenous path. It means there happens to be some other focus of tuberculous in body. These lesions consist of erythematous pepules which become necrotic in centre. They heal by leaving behind a hyperpigimented and pitted scars. They appear suddenly and are heald within 2-3 weeks. A continuous cycling of eruptions and healing goes on from few months to years. Extremities are the common site for their occurrence.

TUBERCULOSIS OF SKELETAL SITES

Skeletal tuberculosis in always secondary, the primary foci being either in the lungs, lymph nodes or gastro-intestinal tract. It occurs mostly in the first three decades of age, however, no age is immune.

Tuberculosis of bones and joints, spine, hip, knee, foot, elbow, hand, shoulder are the major sites of infection. Tuberculosis of bones and joints is not uncommon, especially in children. Tuberculosis of spine, next followed by tuberculosis of hip and knee and with much less frequency of tuberculosis of other joints are the distributed patterns of skeletal tuberculosis.

Skeletal tuberculosis is a specialised branch for orthopaedicians, yet homoeopathy can ameliorate the condition, even surgical orthopaedic cases can be treated and cured by homoeopathy.

Osteoarticular tuberculosis lesions develop from primary focus (lungs, tonsils, mesentery, mediastinum). Then Bacillaemia occurs, thereafter through the arteries and veins, they reach the skeletal system and finally tubercle develops.

Some important factors regarding this type of tuberculosis are as under—

1. Tuberculous bacillus involved in Human, more commonly, but it may be Bovine also though very rare
2. It is always secondary
3. Spreads to bones through blood, lymphatic spreading and directly
4. If the subject is anaemic, weak and ill-nourished and has the tubercular diathesis, it is a predisposing factor
5. Local trauma is also predisposing. The general symptomatology of skeletal tuberculosis is :

1. Low grade fever
2. Lassitude in afternoon

3. Loss of appetite
4. Loss of weight
5. Night sweating
6. Anaemia
7. Tachycardia
8. Evening rise of temperature
9. Pain dull aching and chronic in nature in joints
10. Nightly aggravations
11. Muscular spasms
12. Restricted joint movement wants to stand still and, on examination, tries that no pain be experienced on external rotation—an internal resistance or freedom of muscle is experienced by physician
13. Regional lymph node enlarged
14. Gross limb muscle wasting
15. Abscess formation
16. Sinus formation
17. Pain and swelling
18. Deformities
19. Destruction
20. Loss of joint.

All symptoms can be cured by any homoeopathist easily. The caution is, that, if the stage has reached the disorganizational state, the maintenance therapy of homoeopathy is required. Radiological examination, CT scan, USG, M. R. I., blood investigations, Tuberculin test and histopathological examinations are carried out for assessing the pathological stage.

The utility of classical homoeopathic medicines, nosodes and direct energy medicines (X-ray, Rad, bromatum) is indispensable in skeletal tuberculosis.

Following is a list and brief description of affected sites of tuberculosis of skeleton.

TUBERCULAR OSTEOMYELITIS

It occurs in any of the long tubular bones. The patient complains of pain in affected bone. Swelling and tenderness are seen. Cold abscess or sinus formation and enlargement of regional lymph nodes are seen.

When the metacarpals and metatarsals are involved, this is called tuberculosis dactylitis. Hand is more frequently involved than foot. In phalanges, it is uncommon after the age of five years.

TUBERCULOSIS OF SPINE

It is gradual in onset. It is most common and most severe form of skeletal tuberculosis. It is haematogenous in origin. The leading symptoms of this tuberculosis are :

1. Emaciation, loss of weight, pain, weakness, anorexia, night sweats, pyrexia
2. Aching character of pain

3. Stiffness of back, hunchback
4. Angular curvature of spine. If the patient is child, the possibility of Pott's disease should also be thought.
5. Formation of an abscess
6. Weakness of one foot
7. Dragging of legs
8. Wasting of spinal muscles and back muscles.

In young children acute condition such as poliomyelitis and osteomyelitis produce the same symptoms, therefore it should be checked with great care. Congenital spine disease may also be there.

In young adult's Schmorld's disease and Scheuerman's disease, spondylitis, osteophytic growth, Carcinoma and neoplasm have similar symptoms.

In advanced stage, onset of paraplegia may occur.

This disease is more actively progressing and destructive in nature. Bone destruction is common in advanced stage. Lumbo-sacral, Lumbar-spine, Dorso-lumbar, Lower and mid dorsal, upper dorsal and cervical sites are commonly affected sites.

For homoeopathist, the name of disease is not important. The leading character of this type of tuberculosis is continuous progression, destruction, necrosis and repairs.

If the similar symptom pattern occurs in any other disease, still, the medicines of homoeopathy, selected on basis of manifesting symptoms, work. This is the greatest benefit in homoeopathy. If the case is accurately diagnosed or otherwise, the medicines selected on symptom pattern will act in every condition. For bone destruction of spine region, there are excellent medicines in homoeopathy, which can avert the surgical needs.

TUBERCULOSIS OF THE HIP

Mostly children are victims of this type of tuberculosis. It is also haematogenous in origin. In this, irritation of joint occurs. The synovitis is seen. Tuberculosis of the hip most often starts from a small triangular area on the inner side of the femoral neck just below the epiphyseal cartilage. The leading symptoms are :

1. Joint irritation, pain
2. Femoral bone destruction
3. Synovitis
4. Limb becomes held in abduction and external rotation
5. Muscular spasm
6. Slight displacement of femor
7. Lordosis
8. Deformation of the knees
9. Decalcification of bone
10. Pain in night is stitching in character; swelling, knee pain
11. The limitation of limb movement develops and patient limps
12. Early wasting of gluteal muscle is a strong indication
13. Septic infection may occur.

Tuberculosis of hip is gradual in onset and usually confused with transient infective arthritis, osteochondritis and slipping of femoral head.

In all the above similar pattern, in tuberculosis of hip the above symptom may be there. A homoeopathic medicine will act in any of the cases, if it has been selected properly. If there is a mistake in diagnosis even then the homoeopathic medicine works for similar symptoms. Tuberculin test is a pathological confirmation. Children mostly present the similar symptoms in osteochondritis (Perthe's disease) and tuberculosis of hip. Pathological anti T.B body test and M.R.I distinguishes the case of tuberculosis or otherwise.

TUBERCULOSIS OF THE KNEE

This is gradual in onset. Synovial changes predominate. Destruction of cartilage takes place. In primary stages no movement is restricted but ultimately if disease advances, both in child and adult, the deterioration and loss of joint occur. There is a spread of pannus from the periphery of the articular cartilage over the cartilage.

The leading symptoms are :

1. Pain
2. Swelling
3. Loss of movement
4. Flexion deformity
5. Gross backward displacement of the tibia on the femur
6. Synovitis
7. Inflammation of joint as occures in other forms of skeletal tuberculosis
8. Tonsils may be there.

The common association of pulmonary tuberculosis with tuberculosis of knee has been watched.

The constitutional treatment is same as in other skeletal tuberculosis ailments. It should be seen in conjunction with Rheumatic arthritis where pain and swelling are there, but it is rapid in onset.

TUBERCULOSIS OF THE ANKLE AND FOOT

It is a haematogenous tuberculosis. Peripheral joints are involved. Ankle, Mid-tarsal joint, Sub-astragalonid joint, Astragalo-scaphoid joint, are the major sites. In infants meta-tarsal bones are mostly affected. It is gradual in onset.

The leading symptoms are :

1. Localized swelling
2. Painful swollen feet
3. Necrosis and destruction.

Presence of abscess, sinuses and association with pulmonary diseases are there.

TUBERCULOSIS OF SHOULDER

The tubercular lesion appears in the head of the humerus. A high percentage of associated lesions has been found with tuberculosis of the shoulder, chief of which was pulmonary tuberculosis.

The leading symptoms are :

1. Gradual onset of pain
2. Stiffness of the shoulder
3. Limitation of movement is general
4. Marked wasting of deltoid
5. Pain is a prominent symptom
6. Cold abscess formation is common.

In advanced stage, deformity restricts the movement of joint. Destruction and deformity occurs.

TUBERCULOSIS OF THE ELBOW

Synovitis recurs. Destruction occurs in advanced stage of bony articular ends of humerus and ulna and radius. Tubercular cavitation and caseation occur.

TUBERCULOSIS OF THE WRIST

It usually occurs in the carpometacarpal range of joints. There is a high incidence of associated haematogenous tuberculous lesions. The carpal bones and wrist jonts are the site of infection.

SACRO-ILIAC ,TUBERCULOSIS

The disease occurs in young adult patients. It is a most severe form of skeletal tuberculosis. Lower part of the sacro-iliac joints are affected. There may, however, be a combined tuberculosis of the lumbo-sacral and sacro-iliac joints in which upper joints are affected. Bone destruction occurs. Abscess formation is often there.

The leading symptoms are.:

1. Low back pain
2. Sciatic character of pain
3. Gluteal wasting
4. Wasting of thigh
5. Tenderness on pressure over the joint
6. Progressive bone destruction.

TUBERCULOSIS OF THE CIRCULATORY SYSTEM

Myocardium (muscular mass of the heart) Endocardium (the living membrane covering heart) Pericardium (the fibrous membrane covering the heart) and arteries are the organic sub-systems which may be infected by tuberculosis.

In the lungs and other organs attacked by tuberculosis, the arteries are involved in acute infiltration, Thrombosis and haemorrhage may develop in arteries. In remaining other organs as stated above, the manifested symptoms are as have been described in common symptoms of tuberculosis with additional feature of affecting structural–functional activities.

TUBERCULOSIS OF SEROUS MEMBRANE

In this, tuberculosis of pleura or peritoneum, or more chronic cases with exudation into both the above referred membranes and ulceration or pleuroperitoneal affection involving hard tubercles and thickened membranes may be found.

In tuberculosis of pleura chest pain, which increase by cough or inspiration, localized tenderness of chest wall, rise in temperature effusion, malaise, toxaemia are manifested. Tubercular pleurisy later on is developed with pulmonary tuberculosis and miliary tuberculosis may also be developed. In advanced case, deep organic changes of destruction, inflammation and suppuration are observed.

Tuberculosis of ***pericardium*** and ***peritoneum*** may also be observed. Tuberculosis of pericardium has same general symptoms.

Tuberculosis of peritoneum has fever, abdominal tenderness, tympanitis, ascites, sometimes sub-normal temperature and association with neoplasms as major symptoms. Other pathological symptoms of destruction, certainly, are there. For homoeopathists the treatment of pulmonary tuberculosis along with other manifested symptom is most in these type of cases.

Bryonia is the major medicine of serous membrane tuberculosis along with other constitutional remedies.

8 Tuberculosis in Children

Tuberculosis in children is not a rare incident..Tubercular parentage, or dyscrasia, influences the course and prognosis of a large number of infantile illness. Diseases of lungs, brain and bowel of children are due to this exposure.

Infection in childhood normally takes place either by way of the respiration or the alimentary tract and more rarely through an abrasion of the skin. For most children infection comes from unknown source but exposure and close contact with an open case of pulmonary tuberculosis increases the risk of getting infection.

Many children become infected by the germ of tuberculosis with the formation of a primary focus but they do not manifest disease and some of them show a developed stage of disease. When primary infection takes place, general constitutional changes of fever, anorexia, general lassitude and cough; however, in some cases, no clinical condition is seen except some general reactions.

The primary lesion develops at the site of entry of the bacillus and early involvement of lymph channels and lymph nodes is seen. In post-primary phase, tubercle bacilli are discharged into blood-stream and small foci in various other organ come in existence. Later on, these foci become active and give rise to lesions in bones, cervical glands, kidneys, spleen, brain and lungs and acute miliary tuberculosis with or without involvement of meninges. Respiratory and Non-respiratory — both the tuberculosis may be found in children.

In primary complex, any part of pleura in lung is affected, hilar lymph node shows caseation, spread is rapid along the lymphatics, lesions are exudative, little fibrosis is there and, finally, healing occurs by resolution or calcification and fibrosis. This whole process goes on without symptoms, sometimes fever may occur, sometimes erythema nodosum and pleural effusion mark the occurrence of primary complex.

If child is without appetite, and has fever without any apparent cause and has a positive tuberculin test, tuberculosis should be suspected. Glands of pulmonary field may be enlarged. The size of the glands, the activity of tuberculous process and the comparative delicacy of adjacent structure especially the bronchi together lead to complication. The factors of milieu, as have been discussed earlier, has a bearing on tuberculosis in children. Measles and whooping cough have both been considered, has to influence tuberculous lesions adversely.

If first infection takes place by way of the alimentary tract in children, the primary lesion is usually found in the lower end of the ileum. Sometimes a state of toxaemia is also seen. If primary infection remains untreated tuberculous broncho-pneumonia may also develop. Tubercular cavities, enlargement of lymph glands at the hilum and positive tuberculin test shows an acute primary infection. Examination of gastric contents from lavage or vomit and of sputum confirm the diagnosis.

In subacute or chronic form, weight loss, lassitude, cough, dullness, pyrexia, high E. S. R. may be there. These all are the same symptoms which have been described earlier in common indications of tuberculosis.

Radiographic examination also confirms the stage.

In developed state of acute generalized miliary tuberculosis, irregular pyrexia, fast respiration; slight cyanosis, irritating cough, palpable spleen, and enlargement of lymph glands occur. If tubercular meningitis occur, stiffness of neck, strabismus and pain in head occur. Examination of C. S. F. is the main tool for diagnosing meningitis of tuberculosis.

The other associated nursing factors should not be lost sight of when a child is being treated. The children suffer mostly from tuberculous cervical adenitis or skeletal tuberculosis. Tuberculosis of spine and hip joint is more common in children.

In case of skeletal tuberculosis of children a differentiation should be made from **transient infective arthritis** and **pseudocoxalgia, osteochondritis, Perthe's disease.** In tuberculosis, the tuberculin test is positive, whereas in Perthe's disease this is negative, this is the main distinction between the two. In tuberculosis and osteochondritis, both have the same symptoms such as limping, nightly pain over knee, gluteal muscle may be wasting, high E. S. R, but anti-tuberculosis body test gets it confirmed, if it is negative, it is not tuberculosis. This situation is very common in children. Where more than three joints are involved it is not tuberculous arthritis. It is most common in children that one joint is involved and several are affected in this tuberculosis. It has been said earlier that a holistic constitutional treatment is must for tuberculosis. In the same way the treatment of children should be done **Iodium, Bryonia, Tuberculinum, Bacllinum Phos, Calcarea, Ferrum, Sulphur, Arsenicum** and **Silicia** are some of the leading remedies, which are constitutional medicines for treatment of children in this disease.

A brief but very much potential description of homoeopathic medicines for treating this disease has been given in coming chapter at relevant place.

Post-primary tuberculosis generally affects young adults. Fibrosis is marked, lesion lead often to caviation, heals by fibrosis and scar formation. This is for young adults who have been infected in their childhood by primary infection.

Homoeopathically, it is to be watched if children have nothing wrong but are looking tired in morning, irregular pyrexia, may be sudden fever after physical exercise or any mental activities. Even school work, a rigorous exercise or any ride may boost fever and anaemia. Demineralisation in teeth and quickly changing symptoms may be there. Symptom grew quickly, flushes of heat, headache, emaciation, malaise and not feeling well after any acute illness are some other symptoms. Besides it, catching cold very easily and G. I. T. disturbances and diarrhoea may be associated. This whole picture is of tuberculosis in young children. Physician should observe these symptoms, homoeopathist can give near miraculous medicines for curing this state simply by observing the symptomatology.

9 Miasmatic Doctrine of Tuberculosis

From the point of view of homoeopathic science, the disease of tuberculosis springs up from the inter-play of tuberculinum miasm. Experienced physicians and ardent serious readers are well acquainted with the concept of "MIASMS".

The word "MIASM" has originated from the Greek word *miasma* which literally means polluting exhalations, poisons and morbific emanations. Some dyscrasia or object or subject which overshadows the real natural ego (vital force). No person is born absolutely healthy. A latent pollution or a just susceptible stage of vulnerability rests in every human being. They are dynamic disease-producing powers which stain mental, emotional and physical conditions to abnormal (unhealthy tendencies). Now the question arises from where this disease producing power springs up or creeps in vital force, whether it is outside vital force or a part and parcel of the same. Much discussions have been made on this issue. If the meaning of miasm is taken as an external factor or external disease-causative agent, nothing is to be said, but if the same connotes some internal dyscrasia toward particular pattern of symptoms manifested by vital force, much more can be discussed and proved.

For the cause of brevity this word is understood in following points :

1. Infecting agent
2. Cause of disease
3. Germ disease
4. Some noxious emanation
5. A condition or state
6. A predisposition
7. A dyscrasia
8. A diathesis
9. Dynamic morbid tendencies
10. Morbific susceptibilities
11. Some specific microbes, germs.

As this work is not on the concept of "miasms", a detailed discussion is irrelevant but for understanding the tuberculinum miasm, the above points and meanings will have to be kept in mind.

In the modern era, there has been a great controversy regarding the scientific nature of miasm. On one hand, modern homoeopathists understand the miasm in terms of external microbes; they talk on material plane. For the cause of tuberculosis — Mycobacterium tuberculosis — in this light is a miasm (an external agent, microbe, causing tuberculosis). On the other, orthodox or classical men of homoeopathy thought of miasm as invisible psycho-spiritual vital force.

In author's opinion, the concept of miasm is the king concept of whole homoeopathic science, and the truth lies in augmenting both the views. The circumstantial pathogens which excite the inner soil, and after this excitement, the inner tendencies manifest some specific pathophysiological and mental symptom pattern form the core concept of miasms. (For more about miasms and nosodes, readers should go through author's work—A Phenomenological Study of Nosodes, published by B. Jain Pub., New Delhi).

Tubercular miasm, i.e the bacillus, invades many persons, but, the disease develops or the predispostion to tuberculosis grows only in some. Further, in this cycle, on germinating soil, the infection grows by leaps and bounds. This is the whole phenomenology of miasmatic working.

1. A Mycobacterium tuberculosis exists in milieu, but it is not "miasm"
2. A human body, which is free from any tubercular diathesis, is not a miasmatic state. .
3. But when a bacillus invades any human system and finds suitable atmosphere to grow there and manifest some specific pattern of symptoms, known as Tuberculosis, the bacillus is a miasmatic agent.
4. And, finally, when any human system shows the tubercular diathesis (favouring condition to nourish Mycobacterium tuberculosis) and the bacillus grows their and initiates a full cycle of infectious process, it is phenomenology of miasmatic interplay.

Any case of tuberculosis has the tubercular miasm. Either it may be an established case of tuberculosis, or it may be indicating strongly tubercular predispostion or characteristics of tubercular miasms.

Three miasms, psora, sycosis and syphilis remain in human body. In the anals of history of "miasms", psora is the mother, it is the first and original pollution or stigma of imperfect human class, from psora developes sycosis and, finally, syphilis is reached.

Tuberculinum miasm is also called Pseudo-psora. It comprises of the elements of psora and syphilis. Psora is deficiency, syphilis is perversion and destruction. Psora is debilitated and syphilis is full of degeneration and aggressiveness. Psora is normal, syphilis is perversion. Psora is passive and cold, syphilis is destructive and aggressive. Psora is itch, syphilis is chancre, ulcer or bone disease.

Psora is an idiosyncratic state of predisposition, acting as a receptive ground and fundamental cause of tuberculosis, where syphilis completes its work. Psora is manifested by congestion, inflammation, pain and sensitising miasm, whereas syphilis is ulcerative and destructive. Psora disturbs the metabolic process and shows tendency of emaciation. Syphilis shows defective growth and anaemia and disturbs metabolism of minerals. Psora wants stimulants and meat. Psora also preferes diarrhoea, perspiration, urination and its problem increases by cold. Psora is intelligent but syphilis is suspicious and imbecile.

Tuberculinum is composed of these two miasms. In tubeculinum miasm, due to interaction between these two miasmatic state, phthisis diathesis lies in form of seed. On the slightest provocation tuberculosis breaks out of such patients or persons (if they are normal).

Tuberculinum miasm lies in the background of tuberculosis. The grand and identifying characteristics of this miasm, have been underlined in forthcoming description. The study of tubercular miasm guides the case towards the possibilities of tuberculosis.

It may not be an established case of tuberculosis, but if the symptoms or characteristics of any person fall according to tubercular miasm, it, certainty, will break out in the dreaded disease of tuberculosis, or similar symptom pattern. If due to any cure or care this type of case does not establish in tuberculosis, there should not be any doubt, that, in future, the genetic transmission or hereditary message will develop the offsprings in tubercular diathesis, and the offsprings of such type of subject will be highly susceptible to tuberculosis.

The theory of miasm is an unfailing instrument of forecasting diseases or disease pattern in hands of homoeopathists.

Following is a most practical, most authentic and concise and clear symptom-pattern of tuberculinum miasm :

Perspiring head
Headache with Cold, Cough and Coryza
Offensive head sweats
Headache with extreme debility
Knocks head with hand or some objects
Wants to have head uncovered
Meningitis

Eyelids swollen
Photophobia
Granulation of the lids
Ulceration and specific inflammation
Sunken eyes, red lids
Ciliary neuralgia

Suppuration of ear due to cold
Aural abscess
Ear affections on exposure to cold
Ear discharge copious with foul-smelling pus
Earache during whole night

Epistaxis
Catarrhal dicharge thick, usually yellow
Haemorrhage from nose relieves headache
Tendency to catch cold
Nose blocked and breathing through mouth, snuffles

Bleeding gums
Deformed teeth and teeth decay

Clearing throat as if some mucus is lodged
Sweet or salty pus-like taste in mouth
Ulceration of tongue
Lips red
Deep fissures cuts, ulcers in lips
Pale face
Skin smooth
Swelling of face—puffiness
Blocked nose
Sparkling bright eyes
Tubercular face is round, smooth, with thin lips
Malformed teeth
Ulcers in mouth
Face looks charming even when whole body wastes
Recurring tonsillitis
Pharyngitis
Thin chest
Pigeon chest
Covers the chest always, as catches cold easily
Cannot expand chest
Afraid of cold air
Voice deep
Sore throat
Hawks (desire to hawk continuously)
Deep cough
Expectoration purulent, or mucopurulent
Swelling of glands
Dyspnoea on exercise
Chest congestion alternates with headache
Expectoration-greenish yellow, offensive
Pneumonic breath
Pleural pain
Violent palpitation
Pulse : feeble but rapid
Cannot climb stairs or hills
Desiring those foods which aggravate
Desire for salt and stimulants
Breakfast diarrhoea
Swelling of intestinal/mesentric glands
Duodenal ulcers
Craves potatoes, but starchy food does not agree
Colourless, profuse urination
Frequent micturition

Offensive and putrid odour of urine
Debility after micturition and diarrhoea
Haematuria
Albuminuria
Haemorrhage in rectal passage
Nocturnal polyuria
Morning diarrhoea
Cannot digest milk
Worms
Faces slimy, bloody with a musty mouldy smell
Alteration of rectal diseases with chest problems
Leucorrhea of deep thick yellow or yellowish green-colour
Exhausting periods, looking pale
Ringworm, urticaria and skin eruptions
Paperthin nails
Brittle nails
Mole, warty pigmented growth, papular eruption
Destructing nature of skin
Pain in bones, nodular growth in bones
Periosteal inflammation of bones
Aggravation during thunderstorm, night milk, greasy and oily foods
Amelioration in dry weather

To assess a tubercular personality is not an easy task but if the key characterstics are kept in mind, the job becomes easier. Identification of these tubercular personalities removes the future susceptibility and development of tuberculosis in any patient, if he is not having positive tuberculosis at the present time, provided he is given a suitable Tubercular miasmatic remedy. And, if the case is established in tuberculosis, the identification of this miasm directs the right and suitable remedy through miasmatic study.

Key Characteristics of Tubercular personalities

1. Always dissatisfied - abusive, whimsical
2. Cannot tolerate cold
3. Rapid movements
4. Always changeable
5. Extremely stubborn
6. Lack of concentration
7. Careless
8. Fearless
9. Fear of dogs
10. Depletion, drainage and wasting
11. Emaciation, and anorexia (eats but does not assimilate)

Genral Observation in 12. Pale face, but attractive, long beautiful fingers

"Tubercular" personality

13. Sunken eyes
14. Red lips
15. Attractive oedematous face
16. Constricted breathing
17. Headaches
18. Thin chest
19. "Problem child"
20. Catches cold very easily
21. Aversion to artificial lights
22. Nasal, rectal, uterine oral haemorrhage
23. Flow of liquids exhausts him
24. Desires unagreeable things
25. Aggravation in night
26. Amelioration in dry weather

Physiological characterstic of "Tubercular" personality

1. Vertigo at the base of brain
2. Headache (moving right to left)
3. Anorexia
4. Anaemia – fatigued but mentally keen
5. Asthenia
6. Nightly sweats, coughing, dyspnoea
7. Head sweat offensive
8. Moist scalp, perspiring
9. Hair moist, glue together, thin, dry and dead
10. Pustular eruptions on skin, skin dry and greesy
11. Chronic diarrhoea
12. Chronic enuresis in children
13. Nocturnal polyuria
14. Nocturnal sweating
15. Nocturnal pollution
16. Prolonged febrile attacks
17. Suppuration of ear and eye
18. Ulceration of tongue
19. Tubercular discharge : offensive, purulent, smelling
20. Inflammation of bones and glands
21. Growth in bones
22. Pain in bones
23. Destruction in G. I. T.
24. Epistaxis
25. Paper thin nail, white spots on nail
26. Extremities cold
27. Sexual perversions
28. Soft and brittle and painful bones

ALWAYS REMEMBER

1. When well selected remedy does not work, it is tubercular miasm
2. If there is family history of tuberculosis in any patient, it may develop in tuberculosis
3. If any patient manifests any chronic pulmonary problem, it is tubercular diathesis
4. If any person catches cold very easily, it is predisposition to tubercular diathesis
5. If there is a marked tendency of loss of vital fluids through the way of rectus, uterus, urethra, sebaceous glands, mouth, eyes, nose and ears, it is tubercular diathesis
6. If there is abundant sweating, nightly sweating, specially, it is tubercular diathesis
7. If there is inflammation (chronic) and ulceration (chronic), it is an advanced stage of tuberculous diathesis
8. If there is aggravation of any symptom in night, it is a strong indication of tuberculous state (Nightly aggravation element due to presence of syphilitic state. Tuberculosis miasm is also know as pseudo-psora. When Psora gets mixed with syphilis, it turns into tubercular miasm).. The elements of destruction, ulceration and deformity are also due to syphilitic miasms.
9. Functional disturbance of organs in tubercular patient is due to psoric miasm and the structural deformity and destruction is due to syphilitic miasm. Even malformation is due to syphilitic miasm.
10. If there is emaciation, loss of weight, destruction, loss of appetite, anaemia, fatigued status, malaise, coughing, hawking continuously, nightly sweating, rapid pulse, fever in afternoon and evening and gastrointestinal disturbances, it is a very strong patho-physiological symptom spectrum, to tubercular diathesis. In any case, if these symptoms are manifested, never forget to administer, the tuberculinum miasmatic medicine.

Any case which shows above characteristics is a strong indication to tuberculosis. The "tuberculinum" miasmatic medicines must be introduced in such type of symptom patterns. If the above symptoms are clearly perceived in early stages, anti-tubercular remedies will make a wonder, it is a truth beyond any doubt. Modern medicine or experts of allopathic system have also found that the same symptoms exist in case of phthisis. In actuality, the theory of tubercular miasm is a meeting point between homoeopathy and allopathy.

10 General Principles of Treatment

Always remember that tuberculosis is a constitutional disease, therefore when treating any case

1. Take the every details of history
2. Aetiological factor may be in history
3. Take family history; it gives the susceptibility to tuberculous diathesis
4. Constitutional medication is must
5. Pathological medication is important just for maintaining the cause
6. Individualize the case
7. Rely on the posological doctrine
8. Repetition of potentised medicine shall spoil the case
9. Tuberculosis is a continuous process of degeneration and destruction, therefore, syphilitic factor should be kept in mind. Intercurrent syphilitic medication gives a good check against destruction.
10. In cases of tuberculosis, we are not to hammer down the case but we are to sensitize the case with infinitesimal dose.
11. There may be primary or secondary infection. More than one organs or tissue may be missed; therefore select that situation similimum, which will affect the complex pattern.
12. Proper and due inhabitation, nutritious daily routine of simple/clean life is must
13. If any tubercular medicine has been introduced in only case of tuberculosis and following symptom occurs :
    1. Glands of axilla become swollen
    2. Rheumatic myalgia occurs
    3. Other glands get inflamed
    4. Eyes become inflammed
    5. Ears become affected
    6. Headache or toothache set in
    7. Eruption occurs on thorax
    8. Sweating in feet occurs
    9. Haemorrhoidal tumors rise or haemorrhage begins
    10. Sensitivity to cold in head begins
    11. Any skin disease sets in
    12. Glands of neck and ear get inflamed
    13. Any superficial eruption sets in and it follows the course from vertex to foot
    14. If the patient feels well

14. In this condition, make no haste, get it accepted that the similimum is on work. Do not disturb the action. The results will be hopeful in such case. Hammering of symptoms and suppression of symptoms of tuberculosis are the greatest misfortunes for any patient, so never suppress the things in this dreaded disease.
15. Besides Hering's laws of cure, Author has deduced some laws of cure. A tubercular cure most follow that path only. The laws of cure, which are deduced by author for endocrine problems, remain good for tuberculosis.

    These laws of cure are[1]

    (1) The diseased state should travel from within out
    (2) From centre to periphery
    (3) From up to down
    (4) From highest to lowest, and
    (5) From vital centres to peripheral ograns
    (6) True cure should be nourishing internally,
    (7) Pleasing to mind – the inner man
    (8) Relaxing the mind first, then body
    (9) Harmonizing mind – body or body-mind relationship, and
    (10) Achieving mind = body = mind circle in balanced state.
16. In a gross pathological stage of tubercular disease, always rest on lower and medium potencies and if the case is not so worn out, use higher potencies. For getting better results Fifty millesimal scale potencies should be brought into use.
17. Besides medication, spiritual look of life and regular practice of some light or very light exercise (take rest where necessary), balanced diet, cleanly and airy ventilated inhabitation account too much for cure, this is a truth, note it.
18. Homoeopathic medication is an art of balancing the distorted bioenergy. In case of tuberculosis, the miasmatic factor in the deep hidden cause which disturbs the vital force. Anti-tubercular medicines should never be forgotten, as they balance the distorted vital force. Pathological medicines help, but they cannot take the place of constitutional treatment. Our fight is not so fierce against mycobacterium tuberculosis but our work is to support the intelligent, subtle, and divine vital force, so that it may stand against any invasion.

Following is a list of commonly used medicines :

---

1 Readers are advised to go through author's another work "Understanding Glands; Endocrinology. The Homoeopathic Treatment," published by B. Jain pub., New Delhi

[A] Treatment of Tuberculosis of Pulmonary Region (Polmonalis tuberculosis)

1. General or specific new medicines for tuberculosis (mentioned later in this work)
2. **Generally used medicines**

Phos	Drosera
Stann	Tuberculimun
Silicea	Bacillinum
Iodium	Psorinum
Acalyphal	Caclarea
Kreosote	Arsenic
Ant-tart	Kali-iod
Bryonia	Iodum
Ars-jod	Phelland

[B] Treatment of Tuberculosis of Central Nervous System

1. General or specific new medicines for tuberculosis (mentioned later in this work)
2. **Generally used medicines**

Causticum	Syphilinum
Phos	
Bell	
Glonine	

[C] Treatment of Tuberculosis of Liver

1. General or specific new medicines for tuberculosis (mentioned later in this work)
2. **Generally used medicines**

Chin	Hepar	Sulph
Nat-S	Myristica	Arn
Mag-M	Phos	Nux-v
Chelidonium	Puls	Bell
Car-M	Nux-v	Lycopodium
Chelidonium	Cardus-M	Myrica cerifera
Lyco	Mere-Iod	Nat-sulph

[D] Treatment of Tuberculosis of Spleen

1. General or specific new medicines for tuberculosis (mentioned later in this work)
2. **Generally used medicines**

China	Arnea diadema
Ceanothus	Suceinum Acid
Lachesis	
Bryonia	

[E] Treatment of Tuberculosis of Lymph Nodes[1]

1. General or specific new medicines for tuberculosis (mentioned later in this work)

2. **Generally used medicines**

Drosera	Iod	Cal Seor
Calc	Puls	Tuberculinum
Sulp	Phyto	Bacillinum
Sil	Baryta-c	Merc
Hep	Carbo-an	Thuja
Phos	Ars	Calc-iod
Fer-iod	Dulcamara	Cistus Canedensis
Kali-h	Lapis-alba	Cal-ioda
Aurum met	Conium	Feriod

[F] Treatment of Endocrine Glands[1]

1. General or specific new medicines for tuberculosis (mentioned later in this work)

2. **Generally used medicines**

Drosera	Phos	Mere
Thyroidinum	Iod	Ars
Tuberculinum	Hepar	Calcarea
Bacillinum	Silicea	Spongia
Nat-mur	Spong	Rhustox
Baryta	Ferr-iod	Crot-c
Bell	Agr. nutans	Aurum Tryp
Cal-iod	Bromine	Apis

[G] Treatment of Tuberculosis of Eye

1. General or specific new medicines for tuberculosis (mentioned later in this work)

2. **Generally used medicines**

Aur-mur	Arg. Nit	Merecor
Bry	Staph	Hep sulph
Calc.	Thuja	Sulphur-iod
Alum. Silic	Kresote	Acet-ac.
Euphrasia	Sulphur	Kaliiod

1, 2 For knowing about endocrine glands and other gland; read author's work "Understanding Glands" (Published by B. Jain, Publishers. New Delhi)

[H] Treatment of Ailmentary Tract

1. General or specific new medicines for tuberculosis (mentioned later in this work)

2. **Generally used medicines**

Condurango	Phosp		
Nat-M	Sol		
Lach	Sil		Lips
Arum trip			
cadmium sulph			
Graphites	Ars Alb		
Lycopudium	Lach		
Mangunum	Crot-hor		Tongue
Merc	Acid mur		
Nit-ac	Baptisia		
Iodum	Plumbum		
Phos			Salivary glands
Nit-ac			
Belladona	Hepar sulph		
Merc	Apic mel		
Hreptococcin	Baryta		Tonsil
Phyto lacca	Iodum		
Cal carb	Cal-iod		
Agar	Sil	Mangh	
Spong	Senega	Phos	
Stan	Merc	Kali-i	Larynx and pharynx
Hep.	Calc.	Caust	
Ars-alb	Apocynum		
Bryonia	Ars alb		
Belladona	Lyco		Abdomen
Colocynth	Puls		
Apismel	Liatris spiceta		
Carbo-s			
Chin-s			Intestines
Tub			

[I] Treatment of Tuberculosis of Kidney

1. General or specific new medicines for tuberculosis (mentioned later in this work)

2. **Generally used medicines**

Ars-iod	Kali-i	Ars-alb.
bacillinum	kreosote	Bengoic-ac
Lycopod	hecla	Ars-brom
Cal	Apis-m	Terebinth
Calc-iod	Canth	Phos
Chin ars	Hamematy	Berb-vul

[J] Treatment of tuberculosis of Genital Organs

1. General or specific new medicines for tuberculosis (mentioned later in this work)

2. **Generally used medicines**

Calc	Merc		Female
Carbo-ac	Phos		genitilia
Hydroc	Scrotum	Graph	
Thuja	Bufo	Iod	Male
Bov	Puls	Kali-iod	genitilia
Thuja	Sil	spong	

[K] Treatment of Tuberculosis of Skin

1. General or specific new medicines for tuberculosis (mentioned later in this work)

2. **Generally used medicines**

Cale	Mere	Nit-ac
Caust	Kali-bi	Silicea
Lach	Kali-br	Ant-cr
Led	Thuja	Sulph
Rhus tax	Lyco	Ars iod
Aur-mur	Graph	Calc-iod
Phos	Psorinum	V. A. B

[L] Treatment of Tuberculosis of Skeletal Sites

1. General or specific new medicines for tuberculosis (mentioned later in this work)

2. **Generally used medicines**

Silica	Drosera	Puls
Cul flour	Phos	Stann
Sulph	Mere	Kali-ch
Rhustax	Nit-ac	Crot-h
Chin	Ph-ac	Phos
acd-ac	Sil	Tabo

Calc	Ars-i	Hep
Stamn	Bac	Tub
Rhustax	Bryonia	Sep
Am-c	Am-m	mag-c

[M] Treatment of Circulatory System Tuberculosis

1. General or specific new medicines for tuberculosis (mentioned later in this work)

2. **Generally used medicines**

Aconite	Bryonia
Spigelia	calcarb
Naja	Arnica
Hippozaen	Rhustox

19. Never, and certainly never repeat homoeo medicines in established cases of tuberculosis too frequently, it may spoil the whole case. The administration of Tuberculinum succesively in 1M, 10M, 50 and CM potency in long intervals will do away the tubercular diathesis or susceptibility to tuberculosis in most of the cases.
20. Sulphur and then after four weeks calcarb and finally after eight weeks lycopodium given in a serial form will better any case. If improvement does not occur raise the potency and repeat these drugs. These drugs generally make a favourable background for any further medication. Now if the patient feels better and the tuberculosis is centred in any particular organ, give that medicine, which is suitable for that organ.
21. In any advanced case of tubercular cavities, Bacillinum will bring in a miracle, Never forget this truth.
22. Pre tuberculous polmonary conditions can be treated by Acid picrin, Bryonia, Dulcamara, Fer. Phos, Kali-carls, Lyco, Sepia, Silicea. These are eight leading classical homoeopathic medicines for pretubercular condition.
23. For tuberculous diathesis Iodium, Phosphorus, Tuberculinum, Nat mur, Cal carb, Cal iod, Ars iod, Cal ars, Iodoformum, Kali-chloratum, Sulphor, Lyco, Nit-ac, Stannum, Fer, Sang, Drosera and Bryonia are the most reliable medicines. Threatened consumption or tuberculosis in active stage can easily be treated by these classical medicines.
24. Stannum-iodatum is prescribed in advanced stage of tuberculosis pulmonalis, but if it seems that it has stopped working Irdum should be given.
25. If tuberculosis has arisen from any organ, it should be treated first, the tuberculosis is to be treated later on. If there is skin eruption or ill-effects of vaccination, any homoeopathic tubercular medicine cannot show its action until Thuja or Vaccinotoxinum or Vaccininum are introduced. If Bacillinum or Tuberculinum are used in such type of cases, the tubercular medicines will be palliating the case.

26. Bacillinum is very efficient medicine for tuberculosis of skin.
27. Tuberculinum can cure and check the hereditary transmissibility of tuberculous diathesis; if a pregnant mother is given this medicine, her baby may be much more safe from contracting the disease.
28. If there is any marked tuberculosis gland, the treatment in such condition should be from inside. Surgical cases or practices are the last option. This is a disease from centre to periphery; therefore, the cure should move in same direction, not reverse.
29. Some patients may have tough piles, hardly curable or treatable; if it happens, it is because of tubercular diathesis. Piles and tuberculinic traits and skin eruption and tubercular diathesis are closely interlinked. The symptom pattern of typhoid or this infection is generally found in tubercular diathesis background. Tubercular diathesis is prone to geni-to urinary function disturbances; sun-stroke affects tubercular diathesis patient earlier than others.
30. Streptocein should be given in cases of tuberculosis when the septicaemia is threatened. If given earlier, it will save from many difficulties. Some other drugs which are useful for this state are Staphylococcin, Anthracinum, Pyrogenium, Echinesia, Carbo, Ars, Lach, Rhus and Boptisia. For septic conditions in tuberculosis, these drugs are highly reliable.
31. If Phosphorus—the leading medicine has stopped working, administer Tuberculinum, it will give excellent results, then switch over again to constitutional treatment.
32. Hepar sulph is a great medicine in case of "Cold sores" in advanced cases of tuberculosis. Myristica has also the same function, more powerful than Haper sulph.
33. Tuberculinum is a kingpin in homoeopathic armamentarium. It is all-pervading. Besides other utilities, it is highly useful for tubercular meningitis and tubercular arthritis, tuberculosis of respiratory and non-respiratory fields and, in cases of children, there is no parallel to this classical gem. Psorinum is chronic of tuberculinum.
34. Teucrium seorodonia is specific for young patients suffering from pulmonary tuberculosis. Tuberculosis of testes, bone, joints and glands in young person is always benefitted by it. Homoeopathists must never forget this medicine.
35. Tuberculinum diathesis may develop tumors of tubercular nature in brain, in childhood just after an acute febrile disease. In childhood the tuberculosis of other organs may develop if there is tubercular predisposition in child.
36. Sometimes, some cases of tuberculosis specially pulmonary affections and other associating symptoms with tuberculosis show a time modality. They are aggravated at particular time. A select list of the time modality has been given previously. In such a situation, the time modality

medicines should be used intercurrently. These medicines should not be given at the time of manifestation of symptoms, but the judicious time for their application is either before that particular episode or after. Preferably it should be after the episode, so that new cycle of time modality may be discontinued.

37. Tuberculinum, Bacillinum and Drosera are the leading prophylactics for tuberculosis. If a person manifests tubercular diathesis, he must be given these remedies for preventing developed tuberculosis in future.

38. Tuberculosis of bone of adults or children having affection of caries (Silica, Sulph, Calc, aur, Flour ac), of necrosis (Silica, Calc, Sulph) of inflammation (phos, merc, phos-ac) of swelling and effusion in bone (bryonia, aur, merc, flour-ac and asafoctida) is equally curable, provided the indicated medicine of above group is followed in purely homoeopathic philosophy.

39. Tuberculosis of bones is very common in children. If it is detected, a time-tested combination can give a very big help — Anthracinum 200. 6 dose, then, Drosera, then tuberculinum will clear away any case of nonsuppurating nature.

40. Tuberculosis of lungs has been remarkably controlled by an alternation of Kali-iod 1X and Canabis sativa 1X. These type of combinations are not classical homoeopathy, but if they prove to be true for checking some ailments, we should take benefit of the same.

41. Tuberculosis of skin must always be treated starting with tubercolinum. Any eruption on skin may have tubercular reason behind it. There may not be manifesting symptoms of tuberculosis except tubercular skin eruptions, in that condition, the use of tuberculinum will be of much help. Various drugs highly useful for this problem, as also have been written earlier, are Arsenic, Aur-mur, Cal-sulph, Graph, Kreosote, Nat-Mur, Phos, Psor, Lyco, Silicea, Thuja, Calc-iod, and Ars-iod. Scrofularia and cistus are just similimum for mostly occurring scrofuloderma. The intelligent use of tuberculinum must always be made as intercurrent medicine.

42. Tuberculosis of glands is easily treatable by these medicines. Following medicines are highly useful—Sulphur, Calcarh, Lycopodium and Silicea.

43. Glandular swelling of neck or inguinal region is there; Mere (if the gland is just at the eve of pus secretion); Hepar sulph, silicea, belladona and calcarea carb (if the gland is to just suppurate); and finally if cal flor, carbo-an, and baryta carb is in physician's eye, hardening of gland can be aborted.

44. Skin eruptions and pulmonary tuberculosis pattern are interlinked; they should be examined in depth.

45. Sulphor, Phosphorus and Arseni cum should be given with caution in wholly worn out cases.

46. If has also been concluded that for tuberculins, administrations of tuberculinum and bacillinim is must and for non-tuberculins, where the disease is not established Ars-iod, Bary-iod, Stannum, Cal-iod, and Iod have special action.

47. If sputum test is positive, Radiographs of lung show shadows or contour disfiguration such as of bones, Mantoux test (tuberculin test) is positive, Sedimentation rate is high, and raised leucocytes and lymphocyte in blood examination are objective signals of active disease. If they associate with common indication, this is confirmed.

48. As stated earlier, one should not jump potencies, and sequential potency posology (administration of potencies) is always safer. Major nosodes to be used intercurrently.

49. Some useful hints for more common nosodes used in treatment of tuberculosis :

Bacillinum	Chronic long ailments with thick expectoration, effective prophylactic.
Tuberculinum Koch	Rapidly changing symptoms, sensitive to meat, sweets and smell of food, perspiring easily.
Tuberculinum Residum	Pale-looking persons. Progressive destruction of joints, Fibrosclerosis, tuberculosis of skin.
Tuberculinum Bovinum	Useful for thin and weak children.
Tuberculinum Testicum	Useful in lower part of the body, where the disease is active.
Tuberculinum Marmareck	Pale person, red spots on cheeks, constipation, pain in bones, swollen glands, itching on skin.
Tuberculinum Denys	Useful for tubercular rheumatism.
Tuberculinum Aviare	Useful in bronchitis, broncho-pneumoneal complications of measles. Acute otitis media and bronchial asthma

N. B. : In Indian condition, Bovinum is useful in warm condition whereas tuberculinum bovinum in cold condition the former is better on no motion, while the latter is contrary to former.

50. When the patient does not respond after using any medicine some medicines like Psorinum, Thuja or Tuberculinum bov. altered with Tuberculinum Koch, Tuberculinum marmoreck or syphilinum induce susceptibility. This situation should never be forgotten.

51. Simple but very important point one who is affected with tuberculosis should be free from any mental stressful condition. Stress can cause greater damage and destructions in lesions.

52. If a child does not use cow milk in any condition, it is a strong indication of activity of disease. Children should invariable and strictly be kept away from open cases, dried sputum and dust, droplets of phthisiscal patients and milk of infected cattles or milk which may be infected with bovine type.
53. The modern chemotherapy uses Streptomycin, Aminosalicyclic acid, and Isoniazide. Some other drugs which are of value are ethambutol, ethionamide, rifampicin, viomycin, capreamycin sulphate, cycloserine thiacetazone etc. These drugs can be potentized and be used as tautopathic medicine for removing any iatrogenic disease in a long-standing case, and even their potentization in LM potency scale may prove good and effective medication agent.

11 Some Common Medicines and Their Efficacy in Treatment of Tuberculosis

A materia medica is the final court of appeal in any ailment. Any disease and the pattern (symptoms) of the same must be happily similimum to homoeopathic medicines.

In this work, where the name of any special pattern of tuberculosis or organ's tuberculosis has been given, it means that if this type of pattern exists, the indicated medicine acts very favourably. The indicated medicine is not a specific therapeutics in allopathic style, but the reality is, that if the peculiar pattern of symptoms (which may be known as particular type of tuberculosis in allopathy) exist, the indicated medicine is most reliable similimum to deal with that situation. Homoeopathy treats the patient, not the disease or name of disease, we should remember it always.

Following is an exhaustive list of those homoeopathic medicines which are most reliable in treatment of tuberculosis :

Actea Racemosa has nocturnal dry cough and viscid mucus cough with persistent diarrhoea. Its chief action is highly useful for insipient tuberculosis.

Arsenicum iod is a leading medicine for tuberculosis. Weakness and rapidity of the symptoms are its ranking symptoms.

Acid Picrin is useful in lassitude and burning pain in and between the omoplates.

Aurum Met is highly useful for tubercular orchitis, swollen testes and painful and neuralgic pain of cord. It is an useful medicine for tuberculosis of male genital tract.

Ambra is the remedy for yellow-coloured whitish cough in phthisis.

Ammonium muriaticum has chief symptom of cold between two scapulas in phthisis pulmonali. Arsenic alb and Arsenic jod are chief remedies for pneumonic tuberculosis.

> It is extremely rare to treat and cure any tubercular patient without Natrum muriaticum. It is emaciating. Ferrum metallicum is anaemic and Kali carbonicum is chilly. Never forget these medicines.
>
> Phophorus, Arsenic and Stannum are the medicines for tuberculous, and not for tuberculinic state.
>
> Pulsatilla is a great female tuberculosis medicine.
>
> Acid Phos, Agaricin, Pilocarpin and Sambucus are very effective medicines to tubercular sweats.

1. Acidum Nitricum is useful for pneumonic phthisis. If there is violent cough it has to be removed by some other similimum.

2. Acidum oxalicum is useful in phthisis pulmonalis subject to condition that there is chronic inflammation of the respiratory mucous membranes.
3. Acidum phosphoricum is useful in those condition of perspiration of tuberculosis where painless exhausting diarrhoea, a great depression, and pressing headache are present. It is workable in pulmonary tuberculosis. It is useful where drainage has deteriorated the symptom.
4. Antim Tartaricum is useful for those tuberculous patients, who contact great ulcers and aphthous lesions. If there is a marked history of chronic catarrhal cough it works excellently. Tuberculosis of tongue may also be helped by this medicine.
5. Argentum Nitricum has special action on chronic diarrhoea, as it occurs in phthisis. Tubercular diarrhoea can be well-controlled by this medicine. It is also useful in phylectenular conjuctivitis i.e in tuberculosis of eye.
6. Arsenicum has a wider control over pulmonalis tuberculosis. Coughing, exhaustion and resltessness at night. dyspnoea on slight exertion are its useful symptoms for tuberculosis.
7. Baplisia has a feverish cold of low type in aged persons. It is a reducer of the hectic of tuberculosis pulmonalis. Bryonia is a excellent medicine for tubercular chest pain.
8. Belladona arrests the secretion from salivary glands and skin. It may be useful in perspiration of tuberculosis.
9. Bromium is useful in violent stitches in the lungs, difficult and painful inspiration and long coughs. Tuberculosis of vocal cords is also treated; when disease has central focus in vocal cord, it is the useful remedy.
10. Borax is useful medicine when there is congestion in lungs and constricted and sharp stiching pain is felt in upper right chest. The expectoration has a sort of musty, mouldy odour and taste.

> Thyroidinum is a great sarcode. (Sarcodes are dealt with in details by author in his work "A Study of Sarcodes, Published by I. B. P. P., New Delhi). It is for those patients who are suffering from endocrine disorders like exophthalmus, or myxedema and cretinism. When uterine haemorrhages associate exophthalmus and then tuberculosis is contacted, it is the guiding remedy. But author's precaution regarding this medicine is that it should not be given to tubercular and hypertensive petient in crude dose. If it is to be given it is to be given in potencies. Repeatition should be made for better results. Pulse must be watched. Its substitute medicine Phos, Iod, Arsenic, Nat Mur, Cal-c, and Spongia are great classical medicines; if substitutes are given to patient it will not be wrong from the point of view of prescription.

Calcarea ars is praisal for chronic pneumonic tuberculosis. In chronic cases its efficacy ismarked. It can be used as inter-current remedy in chronic cases.
Calcarea iod is specially helpful for dark-complexioned emaciated children having

tuberculosis of mesentric glands. Hectic chronic cough with a greenish cough expectoration, diarrhoea of green yellow colour and skin is dry except night sweating.

Calcarea phos is a very eminent medicine for tubercular diathesis. It is most useful for first seven years of life. Craving for unsuitable foods and frequent diarrhoea are the indicating symptoms. In tuberculosis of bones of children, it is a very valuable medicine. Female patients below 20 years of age, who have headache as a chief symptom, are greatly benefitted by this medicine.

Calcarea carb is a grand remedy for large cavities, when the case is advanced. Calcarea carb is suitable for children below seven years. It is suitably specific for tuberculosis of glands and bones. If the child is suffering from Pott's disease, it is highly specific for those subjects. It is also useful for tubercular diathesis in children. It is used in tuberculosis of testes with much success.

Carbo animalies, a sarcode, is useful in last stage of tuberculosis of lungs. Green offensive sputa, offensive sweet sputa and dyspnoea are the main symptoms.

Drosera has special action on yellow mucus which is found in laryngeal tuberculosis. Any homoeopathist treating this type of phthisis should try this medicine. Chronic and malignant cough which produces a grave tuberculosis of respiratory tract is easily treatable by this medicine. It is a similimum to phthis pulmonalis. For its spasmodic and chronic cough, it should be compared with Acid hydrocyanicum, Acid nitricum, Cuprum, Hyscyamus, Corallinum, Nux Vomica, Ipecac and Sambucus. Chronic persistent hoarseness, repeated catarrhal attacks, rapid emaciation, severe stitches in chest, loss of hunger, tickling, and persistent cough are symptoms of great importance. Drosera is an unfailing medicine of tuberculosis of lungs and larynx.

> Ferrum Aceticum, Acalypha Indica, Millefolium, and Germanium Maculatum are prominent blood-medicines used in haemoptysis.
>
> Calcarea carb and Phosphorus, given alternatively, check the fast growing tendencies of tuberculosis.
>
> Patho-physiologically tubercles (depositis in lungs) can be easily affected by spongia, calcarea, Hep, Iod, Phos. caust, Ars, and Nit-ac, Their action can be examined pathologically by well-being of patient.
>
> Arnica, Bellis Perenis and Sulphuric acid are the master medicines in tuberculosis where trauma has been the instrumental cause.

Ferrum has special action for constriction of chest, tickling cough, headache and haemoptysis. Anaemia is also well-marked with these symptoms, actually it is the very note symptom of this medicine in tuberculosis.

Gallicum Acidum is a splendid medicine for purulent expectoration, night sweats, evening fever, rapid pulse, loss of weight. It has a remarkable success in those cases where any diabetic patient has contacted tuberculosis; as it also has symptoms of diabetic syndrome.

Hekla lava is useful in tuberculosis of eyes and bones.

Always remember that the first grade antitubercular miasm medicines are :

Bacillinums
Tuberculinum
Calcar-Ar
Phos
Puls
Kali-C
Carbo-An
Silic
Ars-Iod
Iodium
Stannum Met
Dorsera
Kreosote
Spongia
Aviary

Iodium has almost a very specific action for scrofulous pneumonia, which may develop in a full-fledged case of pulmonary tuberculosis. Glands are also affected. The patients suitable for this medicine are dark complexioned–unhealthy skin having and hyperthermic. Food does not nourish the patient, he/she loses weight constantly.

Kreosotum is the homoeopathic medicine suitable for diabetic's tuberculosis. Pulmonary tuberculosis in diabetes is greatly helped by this medicine.

The cases of tuberculosis has time modality.

Following is an authentic medicinal list of some symptoms like coughing, sweating, fever haemoptysis or other symptoms may have time modality—

6 A.M.	–	Ver. A.	7 P.M.	–	Nux-v
7 A.M.	–	Podo	8 P.M.	–	Sulphur
8 A.M.	–	Nux-v	9 P.M.	–	Bry.
9 A.M.	–	Eup-p	10 P.M.	–	Chi-S
10 A.M.	–	Nat-M	11 P.M.	–	Cact
10 A.M. to			12 midnight	–	opium
3 P.M.	–	Tub.	1 A.M.	–	Ars
11 A.M.	–	Sulphor	2 A.M.	–	Kali-Bi
12 noon	–	Sulphor	3 A.M.	–	Kali-c
1 P.M.	–	Ars	4 A.M.	–	Nux-v
2 P.M.	–	Eup-P	5 A.M.	–	Chin
3 P.M.	–	Bell	6 A.M.	–	Ver. A.
4 P.M.	–	Lyco			
4 P.M. to	–	Lyco			
8 P.M.					
5 P.M.	–	Thuja			
6 P.M.	–	Nux-v			

(The above are first grade medicines)

Kali Chloricum is a very beneficial remedy in completely worn out cases of tuberculosis of pulmonary area. In this medicine, the constitution of patient is perfectly emaciated.

[A] Important trace elements, homoeopathic medicines for tuberculosis:

Iodine – Iodine, as homoeopathic medicine has unique role for tuberculosis

Zinc – Zincum-Met for exhaustion and anemia in tuberculosis

Magnaese – Magnum Aceticum for wasting pattern of tuberculosis

Chlorine – Chlorine as homoeopathic medicine for emaciation

Titanium – Titanium as homoeopathic medicine for tuberculosis, and tuberculosis of skin.

Aurum – Aurum met, the homoeopathic medicine for tuberculosis of bones, glands, skin and liver

Tin – Stannum Met-sequelae of tuberculosis

Vanadium – Vanadium, a homoeopathic medicine for nutrition process in tuberculosis

[B] For raising resistance against tubercular infection Drosera should always be used. If it is used after tubercular nosode it gives good response. Besides, it is a must for tuberculosis of chest, bone, cervical and abdominal glands.

Millefolium is great tubercular medicine in cases of haemoptysis accompanied with violent palpitation. Blood comes out without much coughing. Warm blood sensation, flow in mouth is a specific symptom of this medicine.

Myrtus communis has chest pain moving from left lung to right one. Pain aggravates with coughing. Cough worst in morning and better in evening. This evening amelioration and pronounced evening lassitude are characteristic symptoms of this medicine.

Mercurivs Proto is a very useful medicine for tuberculosis of cervical glands and tuberculosis of tonsil is also well treatable. Dry moist skin, harassing profuse perspiration are the guiding symptoms, but nightly sweating is not there.

Merc-Bin Iod is sensitive for syphilitic orchitis and spermatic cord, useful, very much, for degenerative tuberculosis of testes.

Bryonia for tuberculosis of serous membranes
Crategus for tuberculosis of heart
Solidago for tuberculosis of liver
Berberis for tuberculosis of kidney
Iodoform for tuberculosis of glands
Phosphorus for tuberculosis of bones
Silicea for tuberculosis of chest
Arsenic for tuberculosis of intestines
Causticum for tuberculosis of brain

Phosphorus is one of the greater medicine for pulmonary tuberculosis. It has very marked action on respiratory tract. It keeps down the hyperaemia of the lungs oppression of chest, horseness, hectic fever, haemoptysis and burning sensation. It quiets the cough and moderates diarrhoea. Incipient phthisis is also well-controllable by this medicine. It is curative in intestinal and pneumonic phthisis. It proves to be a similie of blood spitting tuberculosis of pulmonary region. It is deep-acting medicine. Care should be taken to introduce it into very feeble patients. This medicine is suitable for those tubercular patients who grow very rapidly and who are of fine texture with an intelligent mind. In case of right lobe of tubercle affection, it works very fast. It is also useful in tuberculosis of bones also. Tubercular meningitis of young subjects is well-treatable by this remedy.

Pix Liquida is a good remedy for pulmonary tuberculosis where very offensive cough and muco-purulent foul odor substance comes out. If there is pain in stomach and blackish fluid also comes out of the mouth; it becomes a specific medicine.

Phell and rium has morning cough for hours, dyspnoea and prostration. It relieves the cough even in the last stage of tuberculosis when tubercular cavities are formed and oedema of extremities, copious diarrhoea, difficult respiration and profuse sweating occur. It is the medicine which can be hoped to act in the last stage of tuberculosis.

Pilocarpus is a specific medicine for phthisical sweating, when sweating (Night sweating) is a prominent symptom — it is a must.

Pulstilla is suitable for tuberculosis in young chlorotic girls. It may be a good female tuberculosis medicine. Yellow salty expectoration, emaciation, hectic fever, fast and rapid pulse are the symptoms of this medicine. For women, it has a specific action on tuberculosis of ovaries and uterus. Tuberculosis dyscrasia of women can also be treated by this medicine.

Radium Brom is a direct energy medicine. Direct energy medicines (Imponderables)[1] are most potent arms homoeopathists. It has been said that when nosodes fail, these medicines work. Radium Brom which is a most potent "imponderable —direct energy medicine", is unfalling in tuberculosis of bone. When tuberculosis of bones does not respond, it should be tried.

Rumex is the medicine for phthisisical patients who have tough tickling cough and dyspnoea at 2 a.m. Its modality of time makes it a specific medicine.

> Belladona, Kali-iod, Thuja, Nit-ac, Hydrocotyle, Calcarea, Fluor-ac and Psorinum are effective medicines for tuberculosis of skin.
> Chininum-sulph, Carboneum-sulphuratom and Tuberculinum are the important medicines for tuberculosis of intestinal tract.

1 "Direct Energy Medicines" have been dealt with in details in author's work "Imponderabillia : Homoeopathic Direct Energy Medicines".

Sulphur has a great power in checking respiratory troubles. Skin eruptions in tuberculosis are also treatable by this king medicine of psoric miasm. Tuberculosis pulmonalis and tuberculosis of skin are treatable by this medicine. The latter is mostly benefitted by this great psoric remedy. For tubercular patient at the age of puberty, it is not so useful, but its intercurrent use produces similar effects which tuberculinum produces.

Spongia has special action for inflammation of larynx, catarrh, hoarseness, aphonia, and breaking cough. It is highly useful for tuberculosis of larynx. This medicine is also useful for tubercular orchitis. Useful for tuberculosis of testes.

Stannum is a great remedy. Its special action is observed in abundance of the sputa of greenish colour and sweet taste, great weakness and emptiness of chest, dyspnea on exertion. If these are the symptoms, this medicine may relieve exhausting sweat and expectoration of the subject. A sensation of constriction of chest, stitching pain, dyspnoea, haemoptysis and pyrexia in evening are some other symptoms. The sense of profound weakness is chief characteristic of this remedy.

Silica is the medicine which is used in highly advanced cases of phthisis. Pale, waxen, and completely unnourished unassimilated subjects who have offensive sweats (and profuse secretion of this sweat is a guiding symptom) call this medicine. It is the deep-acting medicine. Crawling pain and abscess are found in this medicine. It is highly useful for curing tuberculosis of testes.

Vanadium is a very good tonic for tubercular patients for their digestion. As a tonic, it should be used in any wasting disease; it gives satisfying results.

Vaccininum is an age-old nosode–a classical medicine, used as intercurrent remedy for pthisisical cough.

Zincum can check the sweats of phthisis, it is provided that cerebral depression, chronic headache, malaise, chills, palpitation and profuse perspiration all are found in this trace element homoeopathic medicine. Pulmonary tuberculosis of exhausted persons is greatly helped by this miraculous medicine.

Generally useful medicines for tuberculosis in children

1. Calcarea, Phosphorus, Iodum, Ferrum, Arsenic Bryonia, Lycopodium, Silicea, Sanguineria, Kali Carbonicum are generally the main medicines.
2. Tuberculinum and Bacillinum are indispensable.
3. Antipyretics (for children in tuberculosis) are—Chira, Chininum-ars, Baptisa and Fer-phos, Ars-iod.
4. For cough (in children tuberculosis) medicines are—Codein, Hepar sulph, Drosera Lycopod, Stibinum iodide, Cal carb, Stannum.
5. For Haemoptysis—Phosphorus, Geranium maculatum, Acalypha-indica.
6. For nightly sweating—China, Silicea, Iodine, pilocarpus, Agaricin, Adropin, Phos-ac.
7. For emaciation—Iodum, Nat-mur.
8. For diarrhoea—Phos-ac, Ars-iod, Pulsatilla, Nux vomica, Kreosote
9. For tuberculous laryngitis—Spongia, Causticum

10. For septicaemic stage—Anthracinum, Bapt, Arsenic Pyrogenium, Echinesia

For other symptoms in children, the remedies are those which are referred in this work elsewhere.

As such, there is no distinction of paediatric medicine. The same medicine may be useful in adult type tuberculosis. For respiratory and non-respiratory tuberculosis the medicines are common to both i.e. adults and infants. The above given paediatric medicines just expose the general utility of miraculous homoeopathic medicines.

12 Nosodes and Tuberculosis

A noted homoeopathist P. Sehmidt says : "Application of an alternated dose of a pathogenous product for causing the disease of which it is the result form the isopathic remedies, and if it is used after having been experimented on a healthy man it becomes a nosode". Nosodes are the powerful guided missiles in hands of homoeopathists.[1] The drug stock of nosodes come from human pathological secretions or diseased tissues. To be more precise, it will be better to know that nosodes can also be prepared from pathological exudates of animals and vegetables also. But, here we will not go in details, for the unnecessary expansion of subject will be irrelevant, but we should know that they are biotherapies which are derived from diseased tissues, organs or pathological secretions of living organisms. They can also be prepared out of the products of bacteria, virus or other microbes and for their culture.

Nosodes are highly helpful remedies in those cases where a history of "not well since", "non-functioning of any other medicine", "the trends of defective phagocytosis", "the requirement of the very medicine which will pierce deep down the miasmatic layers" and "the acute or chronic infections" exist.

Tuberculosis is a deep infection. The syphilitic trend occurring in this dreadful disease is fatal to life and damaging to vital centres. Our homoeopathic physicians come in stage of helplessness when they find that well-selected classical homoeopathic age-old remedies do not work in a tubercular case. In such a situation, "Nosodes" can work miraculously.

The cases of tuberculosis which are just in beginning stage can certainly be well cured by nosodes. Our master remedies like Tuberculinum, Bacillinum, Psorinum, and Pyrogenium are our prides in treating the causes of this disease.

Nosodes, in tuberculosis treatment, should be given in high and higher potencies (The theory of Nosodes also advocates administration of Nosodes in higher potencies) but, at the same time, if the tubercular case has advanced and the seat of disease is too deep with reference to almost worn out status of vital force, they must not be administered too frequently. In such a situation, a physician, should wait for the right moment, when the status of human vital force allows. But it is, at the same time, true beyond any doubt that an intelligent and judicious use of "Nosodes" may treat any case of tuberculosis.

Following is a list of some select nosodes which have higher affinity to tubercular characteristics and pattern of these symptoms.

---

1 For a detailed account of Nosodes, readers are advised to read author's work "A Phenomenological Study of Nosode" (Published by B. Jain Publishers, New Delhi)

AVIARY

1. Asthenia
2. Anorexia
3. Emaciation—Broken-down condition
4. Frontal headache
5. General Malaise
6. Sensation of chill
7. Myalgia
8. Hoarseness
9. Pain and congestion in lungs and pleura
10. Dry and painful cough.
11. Sneezing and hypersecretion.
12. Congested conjunctiva
13. Pulmonary congestion

Specific for—

1. Beginning of tuberculosis
2. Pulmonary tuberculosis
3. Tuberculosis of eye
4. Special action pattern for respiratory apparatus
5. Tuberculosis of bones

BACILLINUM

1. Always moving
2. Frequent chills
3. Melancholia
4. Violent deep headache
5. Fean of dogs (black dogs)
6. Restless at night
7. Disposition to catch cold
8. Sore throat
9. Chronic cough and muco-purulent expectoration
10. Night sweats
11. Rales of mucopurulent expectoration
12. But very little expectoration occurs
13. Emaciation
14. Pulmonary abscess and Bronchiectasis

Specific for—

1. Where there is hereditary characteristics of tuberculosis
2. Tubercular diathesis
3. Primary complex in children
4. Primary infection in adults

5. Tubercular laryngitis
6. Pulmonary tuberculosis
7. Male genital tuberculosis
8. Tuberculosis of mesentric glands
9. Tuberculosis of intestines
10. Tuberculosis of glands, joints, skin and bones

BACILLUS NO. 7

1. Denutritional state
2. Psychical and mental weakness
3. Tense and tired, pale face
4. Gastrointestinal flatulence
5. Insomnia
6. Polyarticular pains of the back, neck and wrist
7. Pain in knees, Lumbago
8. Very sensitive to cold

Specific for—

1. Tubercular condition
2. Tuberculosis of skeletal organs
3. Endocrine disorders (Thyroid gland tuberculosis)

CARCINOSIN

1. Whimsical, Melancholia
2. Predisposition to pulmonary affections, whooping cough
3. Insomnia
4. Desires travelling

Specific for—

1. When the other homoeopathiç medicines do not work, it is the medicine
2. Tubercular condition
3. Chronic tuberculosis
4. Brittle bones

DIPTHERINUM

1. Rapidly progressive weakness
2. Paleness
3. Anorexia
4. Chilliness
5. Palpitation
6. Subfebrile state
7. Spasmodic cough

Specific for—
1. The tubercular predispositions
2. Larryngal and vocal chord tuberculosis
3. The tubercular affections of respiratory tract

DYSENTERY

1. Nervous and restless mind
2. Irregular sleep
3. Pale colour of face and body
4. Tuberculine personality
5. Pleural pain and constriction
6. Spasmodic cough
7. Inflammation in eyelids
8. Inflammation of nasal; ocular and pharyngeal membranes, conjunctivitis
9. Articular pain
10. Bronchitis, pharyngits and pleurisy pattern of symptoms

Specific for—
1. Tuberculine diathesis
2. Respiratory tuberculosis in beginning
3. Tuberculosis of eye
4. Skeletal tuberculosis

MALARIA

1. General weakness
2. Paleness
3. Troubled sleep with restlessness
4. Pulmonary cough
5. Febrile state
6. Perspiration and chilliness
7. Pain in the limbs and back

Specific for—
1. Pre-tubercular state
2. Beginning of tuberculosis
3. Tuberculine characteristics in any disease

MALLEINUM

1. Worn-out constitution
2. Cough and bronchial problems of congestion
3. Congestion and ulceration in nasal path
4. Syphilitic—destructive tendencies

Specific for—
1. Syphilitic tendencies
2. Consumptive state of advanced stage
3. Tuberculosis of Nose

MORBILLINUM

1. Subfebrile state
2. Diffused bronchial rales
3. Catarrh of the nose, cough
4. Lachrymation
5. Conjunctivitis

Specific for—
1. Primary infection of tuberculosis
2. Tuberculosis of eye
3. Tuberculosis of glands

OSCILLOCOCCINUM

1. Anxiety
2. Sensitive to atmospheric changes, cold
3. Fixed ideas, obsession
4. Does not want to touch others' hands
5. Bruised sensation
6. Chilliness
7. Headache
8. Muco-purulent cough
9. Nasal voice and obstruction
10. Laryngo-tracheo-bronchial congestion
11. Turbid deep colour urine
12. Painful micturition

Specific for—
1. Tuberculin personalities
2. Respiratory tuberculosis
3. Tuberculosis of genito-urinary organs

PERTUSSINUM

1. Restlessness
2. Anxiety
3. Asthenia
4. Sub-febrile state
5. Tracheo-bronchietic adenopathy

6. Whooping cough
7. Spasmodic laryngitis

Specific for—
1. Pretubercular diathesis
2. Beginning of pulmonary tuberculosis

PNEUMOCOCCINUM

1. Anxiety
2. Depressive conditions
3. Does not want to go outside
4. Cough without expectoration in night

Specific for—
1. Tuberculinosis
2. Pre tubercular condition
3. Respiratory tuberculosis

PSORINUM

1. Great sensitivity to cold, sad and hungry
2. Wants warm clothing
3. Allergies and hay fever syndrome
4. Alternate asthma and eczema
5. Yellowish-Green coughing
6. Sticky mucus
7. Chronic ophthalmia
8. Eyelids swollen
9. Dirty skin, sweating and eruptions

Specific for—
1. Tuberculine status
2. Tuberculosis of skin
3. Tuberculosis of eyes
4. Where tuberculinic state is to set in

PYROGENIUM

1. Rapid pulse
2. Foetid breath
3. Restlessness
4. Insomnia
5. Dysrhythmia in sensations of chills
6. Hawks putrid cough
7. Bruised pain

8. Infectious stage of blood
9. Septicemia, Toxaemia and Pyrexia

> *Specific for—*
> 1. Tuberculine diathesis
> 2. Miliary tuberculosis
> 3. Some advanced stage of pulmonary tuberculosis
> 4. Tuberculosis with cavity

SYCOTIC

1. Paleness
2. Anaemia
3. Worn-out condition
4. Night sweats at head
5. Lips dry and fissured
6. Ulcerated, cracked painful tongue
7. Heavy coughing in morning
8. Ovarian inflammation
9. Pain in ocular globes, conjunctivitis

> *Specific for—*
> 1. Tubercular conditions
> 2. Tuberculosis of lips
> 3. Tuberculosis of tongue
> 4. Tuberculosis of ovary
> 5. Tuberculosis of eye

TUBERCULINUM

1. Desire to travel, suffocation, anxiety
2. Fear of dogs
3. Great sensitivity to cold
4. Alternation of mental and pulmonary troubles
5. Chronic headache
6. Irritating cough in evening
7. Sore throat
8. Green fetid pus from nose
9. Nasal passage inflammation
10. Night sweats
11. Insomnia

> *Specific for—*
> 1. Tubercular miasm
> 2. Any tubercular condition

3. A great remedy to be used intercurrently in almost every case of tuberculosis
4. Tuberculosis pulmonalis
5. Tuberculosis of bones, joints and cartilages

VARIOLINUM

1. General fatigue
2. Restlessness
3. Anxiety
4. Violent headache
5. Cough and expectoration of viscous mucus
6. Lupus type eruption on skin

Specific for—

1. Tuberculine status
2. Tuberculosis of skin—tubercular lupus

Among different nosodes, the above referred nosode medicines have special affinity in problems of tuberculosis.

Some other nosodes which are worth comparing are—

1. When giving Aviary, one should compare other nosodes like Tuberculinum, Bacillinum, Pneumococcinum, Influenzium

2. Bacillinum should be guided on the same line of action as in point no. one, written supra.

3. Oscillucoccinum should be compared with influenzium, pneumococcinum

4. Pneumococcinum should be compared with oscillococcinum, Influenzium, Aviary, Tuberculinum

5. Pyrogenium should be compared with Anthracinum and staphylococcinum.

6. Tuberculinum is worth comparable with Bacillinum, Aviary and pneumococcinum. When well-selected remedies do not work, this is a nosode for work.

Aviary — which is a great remedy for phthisis pulmonalis — has the similar action pattern in some other medicines such as Arsenicum Iodatum, Sulphor Iodatum, Pulsatilla, and Ferrum Phos. Some other rare and new medicines like Galphimia glavca, Luffa operculata, and Mimosa pudica also have similar action pattern. For better results, in tuberculosis, it should be associated with oscillococcinum and Serum of yersin. Tuberculinum is a worth-comparing remedy when it is introduced in respiratory tuberculosis.

Bacillinum is good nosode in beginning of tubercular diathesis, as described earlier. When it seem that the field of Bacillinum has passed, the intercurrent use of Psorinom gives excellent results. Bacillinum Testium is a very good remedy for tuberculosis of testicles. The organs in lower half of the body, in case of affection of tuberculosis, have special affinity to Bacillinum Testium. The nosode V.A.B. and tubercullinum have also the similar action pattern regarding tubercular condition of Bacillinum. Nat-Mur is also a good remedy in this connection.

Bacillus No. 7 is highly useful in elderly and debauch persons having tubercular diathesis.

Where there has been a history of heredity of cancer, carcinosin act very favourfully. It is worth comparing with Tuberculinum, Nat Mur, Phosporus, Calcarea-Phos, Psorinum, and Arsenicum. When well-selected remedies do not work, this remedy works with its specialities. Carcinocin is more complex than tuberculinum.

Diptherinum is a very good nosode for throat area tuberculosis. It should be studied with Influenzium, Serum of yersin and staphylococcinum. Fer Phos, Arsenic. Acidum hippuricum and Rajania subsamarata are some other old and new medicines which should be given as per symptoms, but all these remedies have special affinities to tubercular diathesis. The tubercular disorders, where catarrh is the main symptom, is a good rescue remedy.

Oscillococcinum can be supplemented well by Galphimia glauca and Luffaoperculata in tubercular conditions.

Psorinum should not be repeated too frecquently — it takes some time to manifest its symptoms in tuberculosis. In lack of reactivity carcinosis and tuberculinum along with Psorinum should be remembered. If Psorinum does not work, prescribe Tuberculinum and, where Tubrculinum does not work, carcinocin will work. Some other remedies which have some affinity to tuberculosis pattern of Psorinum are Tellurium, Proteus, Pencillinum and Histaminum hydrochloricum. These are new and rare remedies but useful in sŭpplementing the action of Psorinum in tubercular pattern of vital force.

Tuberculinum is a queen remedy of tubercular diathesis and miasm. The only precaution with this remedy is that it should be prescribed where there is no affection of any cardiac problem. **Sulphur, Phosphorus, Abrotanum, Drosera, Iodum, Naturm muriaticum, Silica, and Sulphor Iod.** all the classical remedies of tuberculosis find their representation in this great nosode. This is a pivot remedy to start with in any case of tuberculosis. Some new remedies like, **Aqua-marjna, Histaminum hydrochloricum, Indium-met** etc have the affinity of tubercular symptoms to that of Tuberculinum.

SOME OTHER HELPFUL NOSODES FOR TUBERCULOSIS

Anthracinum is a good nosode where, due to heavy infection, septicemia, emaciation, asthenia and debility have been developed by the tubercular diathesis. One should never forget the efficacy of Pyrogenium at this moment. Besides other types of tuberculosis, pulmonary tuberculosis and tuberculosis of bones may be highly helped by this nosode in such a pathological condition.

In tuberculosis of bones, if unbearable pain in lower limb is seen, ***Brucella Melitensis*** may be another good help, apart from tuberculinum.

In a case which is permanently worn out in tuberculosis and asthenic, and the vital force is quite low, ***Colibacillinum*** is a highly useful nosode.

A case which is fully established in name of fibrous tuberculosis of plethorics can be helped by ***Denys***.

Pathologically established cases of tuberculosis of intestines may be helped by Eberthinum and Enterococcinum.

For pulmonary cases of tuberculosis, where there is heavy catarrh and inflammation, and the symptom pattern points out towards an established case of deterioration, ***Influenzium*** can be of great help — this we should never forget.

Advanced cases of tuberculosis brings in decay, deterioration and structural-functional collapse. In such case, ***syphilinum*** should always be remembered. It is not a nosode which can generally be used in early stage. Syphilinum and Bacillinum have special affection to bone phthisis also. The destruction of bones can be checked by these nosodes.

Marmorek, a rare nosode, is highly useful for the tuberculinics and tuberculars. Paleness, emaciation, sub febrile stage and repeated coryza are the chief symptoms. The patients who have very weak defence system i.e. reticulo-endothelial reactions, may be greatly helped by this medicine. The cases of ***fibro-caseous forms, tubercular peritonitis renal, tuberculosis*** and ***tuberculosis of bones*** are treatable by this medicine.

"Knee-elbow position" case and very weak immunity system with tuberculosis of ovaries is surely treatable by ***Medorrhinum.***

Serum of Anti-Colibacilliary, a poweful nosode, is much help in cases of ***tuberculosis of ovary*** and ***shoulders.***

A case of higher infection of bacille in lungs may be helped a lot by ***Serum of yersin. Tuberculosis of meninges*** is also treated by this mode.

Spengler is another good nosode, which has chief characteristics of tuberculosis like paleness of the face, skin, and great fatigued state; strepto-enterococcinum has also the characteristic symptom of asthenia, anaemia and emaciation.

Toxoplasma gondi has marked anemia and asthenia. It has a marked action on primary tubercular infection. Asthenia, emaciation, subfebrile state, palpitation, pain in muscles are some other symptoms in this nosode. As soon as, in early diagnosis, it is found that there is primary infection of tuberculosis, tubuerculinum should be altered with toxoplasma—gondi. This will so many complications.

V.A.B (Ex-B. C. G.) has definitely the tubercular symptoms. Great chilliness and increased intellectuality, persistent asthenia, headache and great hunger are some other symptoms which are in this nosode. This is a good nosode to start with any case of tuberculosis.

Vaccinotoxinom has symptoms pattern of tuberculosis. It is an useful remedy in tuberculosis of eyes and bones. Symptoms such as general weakness, asthenia, restless sleep and impatient subjects with nervous temperament respond well to this nosode.

13 Some Rare Remedies For Tuberculosis

Some rare and unusual remedies employed for tuberculosis treatment are :

TUBERCULOUS PERITONITIS

Exudative pleurisy	Abrotanum
Tuberculosis with morbid secretions	Acidum Gallicum
Syphilitic Tuberculosis	Acidum Fluoricum
Laryngeal Tuberculosis	Acidum Lacticum
Neuralgia in Tuberculosis	Acidum Oxalicum
Spleen-tuberculosis symptoms	Acidum Succinicum
Incipient tuberculosis with sensation of trembling	Agaricus Muscarius
Haemoptysis in Tuberculosis	Allium Sativum
Pleural effusion, emphysema, mucus secretion, excessive dyspnoea and cough in Tuberculosis	Antimonium Arsenicum
Violent dry cough, stitching in chest, difficult expectoration, expectoration of tenacious mucus	Antimonium Oxidatum
Early stage of tuberculosis, afternoon rise in temperature, profound prostration, sweating, fast pulse, chronicity of symptoms, watery diarrhoea in phthisis, hoarse-throat, emaciation	Arsenic Iodatum
Profuse perspiration in night	Agaricin
Caries in bones Deep ulceration of bone, syphilitic trends of tuberculosis of bones	Asafoetida
Syphilitic tendencies in tuberculosis	Aurum Arsenicum
Destructive tendencies of skin in tuberculosis of skin	Aethiop Antimonalis

Glandular tuberculosis with symptom of inflammation and abscess	Anatherum Muricatum
Tuberculosis of bones, pain in joint	Angustra Vera
Auto toxaemia in tuberculosis	Apis Venum purum
Nightly sweats of tuberculosis	Benzoin odoriferum
Useful for symptom pattern in tuberculosis of liver	Berbereinum Sulphuricum
Chronic catarrhal state of tuberculosis	Beta Vulgaris
Tubercular pain in testes and spermatic cord	Betonica
Destructive tendencies of tuberculosis, deterioration of organs	Bismuthum Metallicum
Nightly sweats	Boletus Laricis
Supporting medicine in tuberculosis of liver	Boletus Luridus
Respiratory tuberculosis catarrhal symptom, febrile states, debility	Balsamum Peruvianum
Tuberculosis in lymph nodes and glands	Baryta Iodata
Just specific for cough, fever, hoarseness in pulmonary tuberculosis	Blumea odorata
Tuberculosis pattern of larynx and trachea, profuse sweating, great weakness	Bromium
Chronic diarrhoea, bloody cough and phthisis	Cetraria
Haemoptysis	Cinnamonum
Emaciation, Neuralgia	Cereus Bonplandi
Extreme sensitivity to cold, tubercular affections	Cistus canadensis

Tuberculosis, general symptoms—emaciation, debility, headache, vertigo, G.I.T. disturbances, painful bones	Cobaltum Nitricum
Nightly sweats of phthisis	Codeinum
Febrile state, paroxysmal cough, tenacious mucus, suffocation	Cuprum Aceticum
Intense headache of phthisis pulmonum	Cumarinum
Tuberculosis of skin, dry skin, urinary symptoms, Ascites and anasarca	Cahinca
Tuberculosis of skin–lupus and syphilis	Calotropis Lactum
Tuberculosis of Intestines	Cassia Fistula
Pthisisical emaciation	Cetraria Islandica
Chronic tuberculosis diarrhoea, which is exhausting	Coto-Bark
Pain in bones, Nervousness, Insomnia, Night sweats	Chrysantheum Leucantheum
Tuberculosis of bones, glands, skin and digestive organs	Dulcamara
Bronchial phthisis	Eriodictyon Glutinosum
Renal tuberculosis	Euonymus Europaeus
Pulmonary tuberculosis, haemoptysis, expectoration of greyish pus, exhaustion, debility, constant coughing	Ferrum Aceticum
Asthenic-anaemic condition of tubercular subjects, tuberculosis Intestinalis	Ferrum Metallicum
Haemoptysis of dark coloured clotty blood in tuberculosis of respiratory apparatus	Ferrum Muriaticum

Pulmonary tuberculosis of young subjects	Felix Mas
Haemoptysis and haemorrhages	Ficus Religiosa
Tubercular tendencies of skeleton	Formica Rufa
Renal degeneration in tuberculosis	Fuchsinum
Pulmonary haemorrhage (to be used with Acalypha Indica for better results)	Geranium Maculatum
Malaise, Pulmonary congestion, and tuberculosis of spleen	Grindelia Robusta
Lupus in skin tuberculosis	Guarea Trichiloides
Useful in tuberculosis of bones, joints, cartilage and tendons, severe pain, aggravation from change of weather	Harpagophytum Procumbens
Specific for phthisisical haemoptysis	Helix Tosta
Respiratory expectoration, serous sputum and hoarseness, continued hawking	Hepatica Triloba
Tubercular diathesis	Histaminum Hydroghloricum
Tuberculosis of skin, and kidney	Ichthyolum
Tubercular meningitis, tubercular diathesis	Iodoformum
Catarrh, colic cough and haemoptysis	Illicium Anisatum
Night sweats in consumption– specific action	Jaborandi
Renal tuberculosis	Kali Chloricum
Pulmonary syphilitic tubercular symptoms	Kali Iodatum
Pulmonary tuberculosis, intestinal and renal tuberculoses, which relapse after treatment	Kali Nitricum-Nitrum
Wasting diseases and phthisis	Kali Hypophosphoricum

Tuberculosis of ovaries	Laminum
Tuberculosis of eye	Laburnum Anagyroides
Exhaustion in tuberculosis	Lecithin
Renal tuberculosis	Lespendeza Thunbergi
Tuberculosis of shoulder	Lithium Bromatum
Pulmonary tuberculosis in light-complexioned persons	Lachnanthes
Tuberculosis of bones	Magnum Muriaticum
Beginning of tuberculosis in bones, ankles, and joints. General soreness and aching	Maganum Aceticum
Phthisis Pulmonum	Myosotis Arvensis
Chest pain in left breast, incipient phthisis	Myrtus Communis
Chronic bronchial cough of phthisis	Myrtus Chekan
Intestinal, abdominal tuberculosis	Natrum Sulpho Carbolicum
Pulmonary Phthisis	Natrum Silicum
Inflammatory haemoptysis	Natrum Nitricum
Symptoms of Phthisis pattern of first and second stage	Napthaline
Chronic layrngeal phthisis, bloody mucous	Natrum Selenioum
Beginning of tuberculosis	Olium Morrhuae
Colic and haemoptysis	Oniscus
Offensive expectoration of cough phthisis of middle lobe	Phellandrium

Ovarian tuberculosis	Palladium
Genito-Urinary tuberculosis syndrome	Pareira Brava
Chronic Pulmonalis phthisis of third stage	Pix Ligvida
A specific remedy for very offensive expectoration of cough in phthisis, emphysema, Tuberculosis of middle lobe, haemoptysis	Phellandrium Aquaticum
Tuberculous Insomnia, due to deep and violent cough	Pescidia
Rapidly progressive phthisis with profuse symptoms of sweating and haemorrhage	Pilocarpinum Muriaticum
An useful drug in phthisis	Polygonum Aviculare
Destructive tuberculosis of bones—caries of bones of feet	Platinum Muriaticum
Tuberculosis of intestines	Pulmbum Aceticum
Sweating, Nightly sweating, Febrile state,	Polyforus Officinalis
Sweating in night	Picrotoxinum and Ranunculus Glacialis
Spleen and Bone affection in concerned organ's tuberculosis	Robia Tinctorum
Insomnia, dry cough in phthisis pulmonalis	Scopolaminum Hydrobromidum
Incessant cough, profuse night sweat and emaciation in pulmonary tuberculosis	Silphion Cyrenaicum
Phthisis-Advanced stage	Stannum Iodatom
Pulmonary tubercular diathesis	Sanguineria Canidensis
Pulmonary haemoptysis and repeated colds of tuberculosis	Solidgoo Virgavrea

Affection of bone T.B., specially of femur, restless at night, great sensitivity to cold	Strontium Carbonicum
Tuberculosis of skin	Taxus Baccata
Tuberculosis of lungs, glands, bone and urogenitals in young subjects	Teucrium Scordonia
Tuberculosis of endocrine glands, exhaustion, nightly sweats	Thallium
Tubercular syndrome of wrists, ankles, and associated cartilages	Trimethylaminum
Degenerative condition of tuberculosis of liver	Vanadium Metallicum
Useful in tuberculosis of tongue	Vipera Berus
Tuberculosis of nervous system	Xanthoxylum Fraxineum
G.I.T. disturbances, constipation, cough and respiratory phthisis	Zincum Iodatum
Profound exhaustion on slightest exertion	Zinc Ars

14 Indian Homoeopathic Medicines and Some Other Medicines

Indian homoeopathic medicines have been derive from indigenous drugs. These drugs have been in use in hands of Ayurvedic physicians since a long time.

When these indigenous drugs were proved on homoeopathic principles, they manifested marvellous results. Though their full proving and reexamining is still being done but the found out results, previously, in hands of Bengali physicians, were amazing.

These Indian homoeopathic medicines are generally used in mother tincture dose. Gross emergent pathological situation are well treatable by these remedies.

In cases of tuberculosis, as such, there is no "specific medicine" from the armamentarium of these remedies, but, as per symptom pattern, they prove to be specific for particular patterns. This is the mystery of success of these drugs.

"Pulmonary tuberculosis" symptom pattern is the main area of their action. These medicines have a direct action on "physicals". There is no theory to interpret them on "mentals". Though this is not in consistency with classical homoeopathy yet this approach gives then additional benefit of direct action. In gross pathological situations, the use of mother tinctures of these medicines give perfect satisfying results.

Following is a list of some Indian homoeopathic medicines which is useful in tuberculosis and allied patterns of this disease.

Abroma Augusta

It is a good remedy for alleviating the nightly or eveningly yellowish-white cough of tubercular subjects. Insomnia can also be helped. These associating symptoms of tuberculosis can be tackled well by this remedy. It the patient is diabetic also, it is an excellent remedy for diabetic tubercular subjects.

Abroma radix is other Indian remedy which may be useful in tuberculous salpingitis. Female uterime disorders in case of ovarian tuberculosis may be helped.

Acalypha Indica

It is a great remedy for controlling the bright red coloured haemorrhage from lungs. Haemoptysis of tuberculosis is easily helped. In this remedy, if dry cough is induced following spitting of blood, and that too in evening, a miraculous power of healing rests.

Blumea odorata

Barking sound cough and hoarseness in pulmonary tuberculosis may be controlled. This medicine may be used as intercurrent remedy for cleaning cough quantum.

Boerhaxvia diffusa

A very rare condition of tuberculosis of liver, i.e. cirrhosis, may be treated by giving this remedy inter-currently in material mother tincture doses.

Calotropis Giganatea

The case of tuberculosis of skin may be helped by this remedy. It is a good remedy for pneumonic tuberculosis.

Carica Papaya

Enlarged liver, in case of tuberculosis of liver, may be treated successfully. It is a good metabolizer. If any tubercular subject finds this remedy helpful for him, it is a good sign as it assimilates the nutritious elements.

Ficus Religiosa

Haemoptysis, haematuria, menorrhagia and metrorrhagia can be treated in tubercular diathesis. For checking the blood flow, it is a good remedy.

Ficus Indica is another good remedy for bleeding or red coloured blood; red means pure red colour blood. It comes from throat or mouth. It possesses greater anti-haemorrhagic properties than Ficus Religiosa.

Justicia Adhatoda

A great remedy for controlling hoarseness, coryza and cough. It arrests spitting of blood. All the symptoms are seen is pulmonary tuberculosis.

Justicia rebrum is another very good remedy for spitting of cough mixed blood. Its action is more sure. Bloody Vomiting of tuberculosis is greatly helped by this remedy.

Acalypha Indica, Germanium Maculatum and ficus indica must be compared when haemoptysis is to be treated.

Ocimum sanctum

In tuberculosis of eyes, where conjuctivitis sets in, this remedy can be applied. It is a great remedy and Indian materia medica of Ayurvedic medicine assumes it as a great killer of all kinds of bacteria and bacilli.

Solanum Xanthocarpum

It is a great remedy for controlling hoarseness with cough. Phosphorus—the great anti-tuberculosis medicine — may fail sometime in controlling these symptoms, but this medicine does not fail. It is a great remedy for the respiratory tuberculosis of beginning stage.

These Indian homoeopathic medicines are generally used in mother tincture dose. A re-proving of these medicines is still under work, but, the patho-physiological situations, as laid in this work, are surely treatable by these medicine. These medicines give a better result when some constitutional treatment is given simultaneously.

Indian homoeopathic medicines in mother tincture dose are a big help to any physician for checking the need of emergent hour.

In homoeopathic philosophy, Mother tinctures are not true homoeopathic medicines, but as they are prepared and used in homoeopathy to palliate the acute problems, and are used homoeopathically, therefore they are considered to be homoeopathic remedies.

There are seven sources[1] of drugs in homoeopathic pharmacopoeia. Among them Herbs, Chemicals and Animals are the major sources of homoeopathic medicines. The therapeutic active agents in these drug sources are extracted in alcohol-water mixture. The potential ingredients in this alcoholic mixture form the "Mother tincture". It is the basic source for all succeeding homoeopathic potentized medicines. These mother tinctures are not homoeopathic but nowadays, they are in use for treatment.

These "Mother tinctures" contain active phytochemicals in case of herbs, complex organic entities in case of animals and active chemicals. As the alcohol extracts regarding "Mother tincture" are direct crude sources, they may have some element of toxicity. In macro-doses it may be a limiting factor in use. However, classical homoeopathic literature shows their wider utilities in different ailments.

As they may have some toxic effect they should be used with great care.

These "Mother tinctures" can be used successfully in following situations—

1. For correcting physiological disorders
2. For correcting pathological dysfunctions
3. For palliating the advanced cases
4. For using as an acutely needed medicine in grave patho-physiological situtation
5. For curing some superficial ailments.

The "Mother tinctures" may have some side-effects, therefore, macrodoses of these medicines for prolonged time must be guarded by close observation.

In cases of tuberculosis, the related mother tincture homoeopathic remedies act on the gross pathological symptoms of human body. This is not to say that they are specific for particular nomenclature of phthisis, but they are specific for the specific pattern of symptoms which are manifested in cases of tuberculosis.

They give the best results when used with constitutional medicines. As a true homoeopathist, we should never forget the importance and potential of constitutional medicines.

In Tuberculosis, these medicines generally help to prevent or check further deterioration of patho-physiological state. In severe cases of phthisis, these medicines help a lot. They act immediately.

The following list of medicines contain some Indian homoeopathic medicines and some others. They are just specific for the situation as written infra.

Tubercular peritonitis and Pleural effusion	Abrotanum Ø
Haemoptysis	Acalypha Indica Ø
Frequent sneezing, Cough, constriction of chest, Hay fever syndrome	Aralea Racemosa Ø
Pulmonary tuberculosis	Arsenicum Iodatum Ø

1 Vegetable, Animal, Mineral, Nosodes, Sarcodes, Imponderabilia and Synthetic drug sources are used to find and process homoeopathic medicines.

Tuberculosis with neuresthenic and palpitation	Avena Sativa Ø
Bronchial catarrh with purulent expectoration, sweating at night, rales in chest, and associated tuberculosis	Balsamum-Peruvianum Ø
Cough with dyspnoea in tuberculosis	Blatta Orientalis Ø
Tubercular leprosy, Pneumonic tuberculosis	Calotropis Gigantea Ø
Scrofulous emaciation with phthisis	Cetraria Islandica Ø
Anorexia, Anaemia, and marked nausea with haemoptysis	Cascarilla Ø
Laryngeal tuberculosis	Drosera Ø
Pulmonary tuberculosis with asthma and bronchitis, betterment after expectoration pulmonary tubercular congestion, cough (should be used as hot water vapours)	Formalinum Ø
Various type of haemorrhages, haemoptysis with tuberculosis	Millefolium Ø
A great remedy for haemoptysis	Justicia Rubrum Ø
Respiratory weakness, difficult expectoration and muscular debility in cases of tuberculosis	Myrrha Ø
Broncho-pneumonic tuberculosis	Solanum Xanthocarpum Ø
Pulmonary tuberculosis	Tussilago Ø
Where cough is a great problem	Farfara Ø
Asthmatic and bronchial affections, bronchial tuberculosis. Night sweats and emaciation	Yerba Santa Ø

Some important observations should not be lost sight of. As "Mother tinctures" are nearly crude medicines, so, when using them, the factor of adverse side-effect should also be kept in mind.

Acalypha Indica, which is a great medicine for haemoptysis, if used for a long time, may cause a dark chocolate colouring of blood.

Solanum xanthocarpum, which is a great medicine for pulmonary and respiratory tract diseases, if used for a long time, may cause unwanted cardiac symptoms.

Tussilago farfara, which is an useful medicine in pulmonary tuberculosis with major cough problem, if used for a long time, may cause damage to liver.

The above precautions should be kept in mind. As a thumb rule, for further safety, the prolonged use of "Mother tincture" medicines must be not made. As soon as they show their curative or palliative actions, they should be discontinued and constitutional medicines must be allowed to carry out their work. These medicines, specially in cases of tuberculosis, should be thought in terms of acute need only. As soon as the situation comes under control, the potentized homoeopathic medicines (constitutional medicines) should be allowed to work.

These medicines are advocated by various stalwarts as Drs. Paracelus, Burnett, Cooper etc. These drugs have special affinity to particular organs. In case of tuberculosis, when the case has become gravely pathological, these medicines may provide relief, they may palliate the case on improve the materialistic working of the organ for some time.

Constitutional medicine finds the true time of action in those moments when these mother tinctures maintain or ameliorate the case. Even physicians treating tuberculosis cases find some time to reanalyse the case for constitutional medicine. Pathological working of these medicines for particular organ is beyond any doubt.

Following is a list of those medicines which have special affinity for particular organ. Tuberculosis of those organs can be helped by these medicines :

Absinthum, Oenanthe, Valeriana, Scutellaria. L.	Brain
Avenasativa, Alfalfa, Solanum. c, Passiflora	Central Nervous System
Cactus, Crategus, Phaselous, Strophanthus, Adonis. V.	Heart
Aspidosperma, Blatta-o, justicia-adhatoda, Lobelia-Inflata, Senega	Lungs
Cardus. M, Chelidonium, Chionanthous, Leptendra, Kalmegh, Ptelea trifoliata	Liver
Ceonathus. A, Helianthus	Spleen
Alteris. F., Hydrastis, Jonosia. A., Ficus Religiosa, Ficus Indica	Uterus and Female genital glands
Damiana, Ikshugandha, Salix Nigra	Male genital glands, Testes
Berberis V., Sarsaparilla, Liatris spiceta, Vesicaria. C.	Renal tract and Kidney

15 Some New Remedies For Tuberculosis

To say the mentioned remedies as new remedies is a traditional concept of course, these remedies are still to be taken by homoeopathic fraternity. These medicines have a vast potential. For the clinical pattern or clinical diagnosis of tuberculosis, these remedies stand similimum to the situation:

ALLOXANE

- Nervousness
- Forgets recent facts
- Spelling mistake
- Lips dry, eyes inflamed
- Lumbosacral pain—Coxarthrosis pattern
- Dry eczema

This is a remedy in those cases where the ***tuberculosis of hip joint,*** specially in children, is found. ***Tuberculosis of skin*** is also controllable. ***Tuberculosis in diabetics*** can also be helped.

The key symptoms of this remedy are :

- Forgets recent events
- Seeks solitude
- Dryness of skin

N. B. ***ANACARDIUM ORIENTALE*** is an old remedy but it is highly useful in those cases of tuberculosis which have audio-video hallucination and ***tubercular affections of Urogenital tract.***

ARNANEA IXOBOLA is a new remedy. Nervousness and myalgia and ***Tuberculosis of skin*** can be helped by it. Dermal eruptions are of erythematous nature.

ARISTOLOCHI CLEMATITIS

- Depressed, weakness
- Abdominal distension

This is a great remedy for tubercular conditious, specially in women. ***Tubercular pattern of genitourinary tract*** can be successfully treated by this medicine.

The keynote symptoms of this remedy are :

- Worn out condition
- Genito-urinary problems

N. B. ***Aserum Europaeum*** is a promising medicine in male patients who have ***tuberculosis of kidney or alike pattern of problems.*** Tubercular diatheses remains in such type of patients.

ASTRAGALUS EXCAPUS

- Nervous unstable subjects
- Dyspnoea
- Respiratory troubles

This is a great remedy for ***Osteochondrites,*** not tuberculosis, but a like pattern, mostly found in children. It is also useful in Perthe's disease.

The key symptom of this remedy are :

- Alternating mental and pulmonary affections

N. B. ***Tuberculosis,*** specially ***skeletal tuberculosis,*** may precipitate in trauma, Bellis-perenis and Arnica are highly useful. In case of children, if skeletal tuberculosis or osteochondritis occur, these medicines should never be forgotten for intercurrent administration. ***Tuberculosis of lymph gland*** is treatable by Bunias Orientalis. The patient (child) becomes emaciated, subfebrile and fatigued. This medicine has a good scope for the aforementioned tuberculosis.

- ***Buthus Australis,*** a new remedy has specific symptom of night sweating.
- Aqua marina is very good medicine in the beginning of tuberculous state.
- Argentum metalicum is a remedy which is useful in tuberculosis of male genital (testes).
- Kali Carb is a very good medicine for tuberculosis of kidney too.
- For pulmonary tuberculosis never forget Beryllium Metlalicum, and Sulphuric Acidum and Lippia Mexicana (adjuvant pulmonary tuberculosis).
- ***Majeptil*** and ***Cadmium metallicum*** are two very potential medicines which have special action for tuberculides. Tuberculosis of glands, male genital organs, heart, eyes and in other cases where nodular tuberculinic focus develop these remedies are highly useful.

AQUA MARINA

- Slowness, torpor and general apathy
- Fever in morning
- Weakness in morning
- Foetid sweats and headaches
- Thoracic and dorsal pain
- Cough, coryza and watery discharge
- Thick mucus, foetid smell
- Difficulty in expectoration
- Sweating.

This is a great remedy in those cases where the tubercular pattern of symptoms set in. It is highly useful medicine in beginning of ***tuberculosis of respiratory apparatus. Para-tubercular conditions*** are also helped by this medicine.

The key symptoms of this remedy are :

- A general and genital weakness
- Thoracic and dorsal pain
- Mucus expectoration

- Rusty taste
- Fever in morning

ARGENTUM METALLICUM

- A highly melancholic personality
- Emaciation, premature senile symptoms
- Desire for fresh air
- Weak memory
- Metabolic slackness
- The patterns of laryngitis and pharyngitis
- Skeletal affinities, swelling of joints

This is a effective remedy in cases of ***tuberculosis of skeleton, bone, joints and attached cartilages and ligaments.*** This has a special action for orthopaedic organs. In cases of ***tuberculous salpingitis*** and ***epididymotesticular syndrome,*** this is a very useful medicine.

The key symptoms of this remedy are :

- Hypochondriac-melancholic personality
- Weakness in chest
- Great hunger and nausea due to hunger
- Feels head as empty bowl
- Palpitation
- Cough from laughing
- Hoarseness in throat and grey jelly mucus
- In males, seminal emission without sexual excitement
- In females, menopausal hemorrhage and leucorrhea
- Neuro-degenerative cutaneous symptoms leading to degeneration.

AGAVE TEQUILANA

- General asthenia and myalgia
- Headache
- Moist cough
- Insomnia
- Erratic rheumatic pains
- A worn out degenerating personality
- Ovarian and testicular pain

This is a great remedy for ***fibrous tuberculosis.*** The other associated tubercular pattern of ***pulmonary*** area is also easily treatable by this.

The key symptoms of this remedy are :

- High desire for spirituous liquids
- Alcoholic tendencies
- Insomnia : difficulty in sleeping
- Polyarticular-muscular pains

BERYLLIUM METALLICUM

- Progressive emaciation
- Sub febrile state
- Headache
- Pain radiating from left mastoid to right one
- Acute coryza
- Dry cough with expectorations of streaks of blood

This is a useful remedy in beginning of tuberculosis. A tubercular status is well-reflected. ***Tuberculous laryngitis*** and ***pulmonary tuberculosis*** are well-treatable by this medicine.

The key symptoms of this remedy are :

- Progressive emaciation
- Capricious appetite
- Nausea on seeing or smelling food
  Clinical pulmonary sclerosis (hardening of tissue of pulmonary region)

B. C. G.

- Paleness of face
- Numbness and acheing of the head
- Great fatigue
- Extreme chilliness
- Depression
- Cannot find the right word
- Violent headache
- Pain in right side of tonsils
- Slight nausea
- Eyes irritated
- Stools (watery or liquid) then change in solid mass
- Great sensitivity of skin
- Chapped and dry skin

This is the remedy whose proving is quite new — it is a suitable remedy for ***tubercular state, tubercular rheumatism*** and ***worn out susceptible*** conditions of tuberculosis.

The key symptoms of this remedy are :

- "Tubercular state" symptoms
- Weakness, paleness, nausea
- Diarrhoea

CHLOROPROMAZINE

- Hallucination
- Insomnia
- Gastro-intestinal troubles
- General weakness

This is a remedy when predisposition to tuberculosis occurs in second spell. Old lesions develop again. In untreated cases and in children, it may be there.

The key symptoms of this remedy are :

- Hallucinations
- Hepatic problems

N. B. ***Cicuta Virosa,*** though an old remedy, is highly useful in school-going children who have developed ***tuberculosis of eye.*** Children show the tendencies of general emaciation and worn-out conditions.

Cobaltum has the similar emaciation pattern it is also worth comparable in tuberculosis of eye. Here the symptoms are of purulent nature.

EXPELETIA GRANDIFLORA

- Worn out constitution
- Prematured ageing
- Headache
- Pulmonary affections, infiltration and inflammations
- Pelvic zone bone problems

This is a remedy when the subject is predisposed to ***pulmonary tuberculosis*** pattern of symptoms. ***Tuberculosis of hip joint*** disease is also worth noting in this medicine.

The key symptoms of this remedy are :

- A sense of always being ill
- Using wrong words

GALINSOGA PARVIFLORA

- Asthenia
- Headache
- Diarrhoea
- Dyspnoea with little exertion
- Acute articular pains
- Sweating

This is a remedy useful for ***tuberculous state.***

The key symptoms of this remedy are :

- Worn out constitution
- Tuberculous similimum

N. B. ***Harpagophytum Procumbens*** is a remedy which should be used in osteochondritis. Where eczema alternates with arthrosis and sweating persists it should be used. It is comparable with ***Astragalus Excapus*** but the situations are different.

HEDERA HELIX

- A deep rooted constant anxiety
- Palpitation and headache, specially of left side

- Great appetite
- Sub-febrile state
- Some endocrine disorders, specially of thyroid gland

This is a very useful medicine for the clinical cases of ***genital organ tuberculosis.*** Associating tuberculous states with genital tuberculosis are also treatable. Thyroidinum—the sarcode — should be compared.

The key symptoms of this remedy are :

- Wants fresh air but takes cold easily
- Voracious appetite with gastric cramps
- If any tuberculosis case with thyroid disease (Basedow's disease of colloidal goitre) is there, it is of much worth.

N. B. ***Histaminum Hydrochloricum*** is useful in ***tuberculosis of heart and genito-urinary tract.*** Genital tract is mostly affected.

KALI CARBONICUM

- Melancholia-Depression, weeping
- Asthenia, fatigue
- Headache in left frontal region
- Headache
- Restless sleep
- Violent palpitation; Inflammation of heart membranes
- Violent dry cough
- Great sweating
- Dyspepsia
- Pulmonary emphysema, dilatation and destruction of air passage, breathing difficulty
- Turbid urination
- Pelvic region pain and inflammation.

This is a great remedy for ***renal tuberculosis*** and ***tuberculosis of thyroid gland*** and ***hip joint and tuberculosis of heart.*** It is a effective remedy, it should be explored. It is a completely tuberculous medicine.

The key symptoms of this remedy are :

- Retention of fluid
- Stinging pain

N. B. ***Levomepromazine*** is an antitubercular medicine which manifests all its symptoms as are seen in any tubercular condition, i.e emaciation, malaise, insomnia, subfebrile state, weakness, night sweating, constipation. This medicine is very much akin to Tuberculinum and Iodum.

Lippia Mexicana is a valuable remedy which is suitable for ***pulmonary tuberculosis.*** This manifests the common indications of tuberculosis. In females where early abortion is a habit and, conicidentally, there is tuberculosis, this medicine will be a panacea.

LOPOPHYTUM LEANDRI

- Fatigue in the morning
- Bursting headache
- Intense thirst and sweating
- Palpitation
- Congestion in thyroid, Dysfunction of thyroid
- Dysfunctions in pituitary

This is a great remedy which must invariable be used in tuberculosis of thyroid gland and pituitary.

The key symptoms of this remedy are :

- Constriction in neck
- Sweating
- Palpitation

N. B. This is a most beautiful remedy which is similar to action on endocrine glands as Iodum, Nat Mur and tuberculinom act. Another remedy ***Magnesium Fluoratum*** has a certain action of cervical adenitis (tuberculosis of lymph glands) and treats ***tuberculosis of thyroid gland.*** It is almost a specific for the mentioned tuberculosis.

NEPENTHES

- Retarded growth
- Fever
- Restlessness
- General fatigue
- Heaviness of head
- Great disturbances in digestion and genitals

This is a remedy useful in left ***hip joint tuberculosis pattern*** or a similar pattern i.e. left cox-arthrosis, which is not tuberculosis. This is also a medicine which can be used in tuberculosis of genital sphere.

The key symptoms of this remedy are :

- Digestion problems
- Genital tract problems

N. B. ***Onopordon Acanthium and Paloondo*** have special action pattern of osteochondritis, a syndrome similar to tuberculosis of hip joint. The latter has a marked myalgia. If any child does not have ***skeletal tuberculosis,*** in similar pattern, these medicines are highly useful. Arnica, Bellis-p, and Harpagophytum Procumbens are worth comparing.

PENCILINUM

- Asthenia
- Sensitivity to cold
- Sub-febrile state
- Frontal headache
- High infection susceptibility

This medicine is highly useful in ***genital tuberculosis of females. Tuberculinic amenorrhoea*** is easily treatable by this remedy. This is a tuberculinic remedy.

The key symptoms of this remedy are :

- High susceptibility to infection
- Intense asthenia

N. B. Like any tuberculinic state, ***R.N.A.*** and ***Psilocybe Caerulescens*** also have the tubercular characteristics.

SULFONAMIDE

- Fatigue
- Headache
- Conjunctivitis

This is a remedy which is useful in affection of ***tuberculosis of eye.***

The key symptom of this remedy are :

- Nocturnal emission

N. B. ***Sulfurosum Acidum*** is equally useful in tuberculosis of eye. This remedy has markedly pulmonary symptoms

SAROTHAMNUS SCOPARIUS

- Extreme sensation of cold
- Troubling headache
- Insomnia
- Congestion of thyroid
- Alternate diarrhoea and constipation

This medicine is highly useful for ***tuberculosis of intestines*** and ***thyroid glands.***

The key symptoms of this remedy are :

- Palpitation
- G. I. T. disturbances
- Thyroid

16 Bed-side Specifics

The concept of "specifics" or "bed-side specifics" has no meaning, if we think over the matter with seriousness. However, the bed-side specifics are used frequently in practice. In actuality, "bed-side specifics" are those medicines which are befitting, to some particular symptom patterns. The manifesting "symptom pattern" may have any name of disease, but the "bed-side specific medicine" is not a response to a particular name of disease, it is a "similia response" to some specific pattern of symptoms.

These bed-side specifics are more useful in following situations :

1. to start with at least
2. In emergency or first aid situation
3. When the whole case is not open, in that condition some medication is better than nothing
4. Where there are no clear indications for a medicine
5. Where the case is to be abridged for some time, after that, the physician will chalk out the whole case
6. Where the physician is very busy and he will look after the whole case in his study time, after his busy days or hours.

Bed-side specifics in tuberculosis, as have been narrated in following list, have a great potential to deal with the organic, pathological and even constitutional necessities. These specifics are not similum, generally, but, coincidentally, if the whole symptom pattern is in conformity with this, these medicines prove to be "accidental similimum".

The bed-side specifics of tuberculosis are not only "specifics" but "simila" also to those symptom patterns which are commonly seen in tuberculosis.

RESPIRATORY TUBERCULOSIS

Tubercular diathesis	Tuberculinum, Bacillinum, ArsIod, Cal Iod, Iodum, Phos, Nat Mur, Stamum
Tubercular inheritance	Tuberculinum, Bacillinum
Pulmonary tuberculosis	Arsenic-Iod, with constitutional medicine
Pulmonary tuberculosis caviation	Pyrogen
Tubercular cachexia	Kreosote
Tuberculosis - fibrous Pulmonary fibrosis	Tuberculinum

Chronic Pulmonary tuberculosis	Sulfurosum Acidum (Sulphur Dioxide)
Incipient of tuberculosis of respiratory apparatus	Tuberculinim, Medorrhinum, Pertussin, Marmorek Serum of spengler
Tuberculosis of the larynx	Cuprum Met, Drosera Sabal serr
Sweating in tuberculosis	Cal Carb
Tubercular emaciation	Sodium, Nat Mur, Phos, Cal Phos
Glandular tuberculosis	Sycotic
Haemoptysis in tuberculosis of lungs	
(1) When blood is red	Ipecac alternated with millefolium
(2) When blood is black	Elaps
(3) With dyspnoea	Arnica
(4) After exertion	Urt-u
General Haemoptysis	Acalypha Indica Q and Geranium Mac Q

NON-RESPIRATORY TUBERCULOSIS

Tuberculosis of Intestines (tuberculosis of mesenteric glands)	Phosphorus, Silicea
Tuberculosis of testicles	Aurm-Met, Spongia, Cal Carb, Silicea, Sulphur
Tubercular diathesis	Ars, Calc, Ferr, Iod, Phos, Stan, Tuberculinum, Bacillinum, Kali-C
Tuberculosis of hip region	Tuberculinum
Tuberculosis of joints	Tuberculinum
Tuberculosis of bones, glands, and of necrotic nature	Drosera
Tuberculosis of bones (skeletal tuberculosis)	Tuberculinum and Drosera, alternately
Tuberculosis of eye	Argentum nitricum

17 Autobioenergy Medicine and Tuberculosis

Regarding autobioenergy, author has given a detailed account of the subject in his work "Homoeopathic Direct Energy Medicines"

Autobioenergy medicines are those medicines which are prepared from the pathological material obtained from the patient himself. The obtained material is potentized homoeopathically and used as auto-nosodes.

The autobioenergy medicines prepared and obtained in this way have extended miasmatic spirit in themselves. Thus these types of medicines are not only similimum to patient's symptoms but also to the acting original miasm. Thus they achieve the status of "similimum".

In cases of tuberculosis or tubercular diathesis; the tuberculosis miasm remain active and on constant work. A patient who is suffering from tuberculosis excretes the bio-chemical secretions or, if he is a dormant case, he has the tubercular diathesis active, which can be achieved in his pathological secretions.

Author has suggested thirty different secretions in his above-referred work. For patients of tuberculosis, different drug stocks which can be used as "autobioenergy medicines" are as :

Blood
Pus and Cough of phthisis
Phthisisical sweats
Purulent expectoration
Sputum
Ovarian discharges
Semen
Tubercular bone secretion.

As we know that the major characteristics of mycobacteriun tuberculosis are :

1. They are gram-positive, non-sporing non-motile strictly aerobic bacilli
2. They are of branching tendency
3. They are acid-fast and have characteristic of acid and alcohol fastness.
4. Their cell wall contains a special waxy material
5. They grow very slowly in artificial culture
6. As chemical compositions, they contain

   Mycol – responsible for fast acid staining
   Lipoid – phosphatids, wax and glyceroid
   Polysaccharide – responsible for necrosis and destruction caseation and tubercle formation
   Protein – responsible for allergy and immunity

We know that tuberculosis has the patho-physiological effect on human body in form of inflammation, tubercle formation, caseation, fibrosis and calcification. These characteristics are formed. The T.B. bacteria survives and multiply within phagocytic cells such as macrophages etc.

When the case of tuberculosis (specially in pulmonary tuberculosis) begins, the first reaction starts by evidence of hypersensitivity to tuberculosis bacteria. At this time the minor evidences or common indications start manifesting in case tuberculin test proves positive. At this time, cell-mediated immunity develops and tubercles (a nodule) are formed. If this immunity is strong enough, the infection process is halted but tuberculous bacilli live in dormant stage and patient looks healthy but he is susceptible to tubercular stimulation. He has tubercular diathesis. If the cell-mediated immunity remains weak, the progress of disease starts by death of macrophages and, in the tubercle, caseation and necrosis develop. Even now the lesions may undergo a healing process called Calcification.

When the autobioenergy medicines are introduced to any patient, they act as supportive to cell-mediated immunity. It happens because in the same miasmatic factor which has allowed to break out a case in formation of tubercle, when treated reversely by high potentization of the same miasm, a booster miasmatic mechanistic dose process takes place. Specially in cases where ***auto-haemotheraphy*** is used, it is more eccentric in its action.

Homoeopathic fraternity can use and make further researches on the auto-bioenergy therapy in the patient of tuberculosis.

These medicines, in case of tuberculosis, may help in following manner

1. By boosting immunity
2. By introducing the exact befitting similimum, and
3. By a vaccination in those cases where tubercular diathesis is manifesting.

They may also be used as a preventive and curative instrument. If these medicines are used, they should be better prepared in fifty millesimal scale potency. They should never be repeated too frequently and must never be mixed with any ex-nosode. They should be used between 0/6 to 0/20. It is, however, a matter of personal experience.

A great possibility of cure of tuberculosis lies in these medicines. For a detailed philosophy, readers should consult author's work on this topic.

In cases of highly toxaemic nature, where major pathological changes have taken place, this therapy may be used with much success especially in some conditions like

1. Phylectenular Conjunctivitis
2. Necrotic and Pus secreting bones
3. Advanced pulmonary tuberculosis
4. Advanced tuberculosis intestinalis

The above diseases preception that major scientific research and publication of research findings must be undertaken for cause of homoeopathy.

18 Some Illustrations

To show the efficacy of homoeopathic medicines, some authentic illustrations are being given :

Case 1 : (Tubercular lymphadenits) Noted, distinguished and respected stalwart of homoeopathy in India—Dr. Diwan Harish Chand had noted his clinical experience of a case of Tubercular lymphadenitis. His patient was a young man who was having a swollen gland in his left supraclavicular region and previously he was having a swollen submental gland. For both the ailments, he received allopathic treatment. After ten years the patient again noticed the painless gland, he took allopathic medicines without any success.

Dr. Chand took the case homoeopathically and prescribed medicines like Tuberculinum bovinum, Calcarea-iodata; and was cured, again he noticed some submandibular lymph node and again he was given Clacarea iodatata and Sac-lac.

The patient was totally cured and under Dr. Chand's medical supervision.

Comments : For full details, readers should consult Dr Chand's magnumopus-Microdoses Megaresults, published by National Homoeopathic Pharmacy, New Delhi. This case shows the most befitting similimum of tuberculosis has been found equallly workable in tuberculous lymphadenitis. One major point noticeable is that allopathic treatment does not complete the cure this has been manifested by this illustrative case. Dr Chand had used his medicines in centesimal scale in medium potency, i.e 200, and had used scientific frequency of posology.

Case 2 : (Tubercular lymphadenitis) This case is again of Dr. Chand, who has treated an old lady who was diabetic. She developed a swelling which was painless on left side of her neck. AIIMS specialist could not diagnose whether it was enlarged lymph node or submandibular gland !

Dr. Chand started his treatment by giving her Calcarea iodata 200/3, then Sac-lac; again he prescribed her calcarea iodata 200/3. For reducing glandular enlargement he prescribed Cal Flor Gx but without any result; then he prescribed her Carbo-animalis 200/3. The case was cured.

Comments : The reference is the same as per case no. 1. This case shows that if it was a tubercular lymphadenitis or a similar pattern on a diabetic back ground and base, then homoeopathic tubercular medicines cured the case. The medicines were prescribed in centesimal scale in 200 potency; though Dr. Chand had ordered the lady to continue the allopathic treatment for controlling diabetes. Even when allopathy is running, homoeopathic medicines work. It is the mystery which this case shows. Dr Chand's method of posology has a superb command on medicine and potency as he does not intend to repeat medicine repeatedly.

Case 3 : (Tubercular affection in Pulmonary region)

Dr Chand has quoted a case of aged male patient who was having diabetes mellitus, left pleural tubercular effusion and uraemia. Dr Chand prescribed this patient Arsenic alb, Tuberculinum, Phosphorus Sac-lac and Iodatum.

Much clinical details and case reports can been seen in above-referred Dr Chand's work. The major point worth noticing is that classical homoeopathic remedies who have tubercular miasmatic action controlled the case effectively. Any homoeopath should know how to control the potential and intelligence of medicine with sense of judiciousness. Dr Chand has also proved through this csae that a case which has gone pathologically in nature and seems to be uncontrollable, can be treated and well-controlled by homoeopathic medicines.

Case 4 : (Tuberculoma of brain)

This case is again of Dr Chand's genius where he cured the tuberculoid in brain which was with another ailment "Secundum Type ASD (IICU)". Readers can have a detailed note of this case in the above-referred authentic work of Dr Chand.

Dr Chand had prescribed his patient homoeopathic medicines like Tuberculinum Bovinum, Silica, Pulsatilla, Heparsolp. All these medicines were prescribed in middle potency range.

Comments : These medicines cured A S D and, as such, tuberculoma in the brain was also cleared. Allopathic surgeon also took this cure as unbelievable.

All these cases show that the general classical medicines which are used in tuberculosis can work an unbelievable result provided they are applied judiciously.

Case 5 : (Glandula Tuberculosis)

Senior physician and most distinguished man of homoeopathic science Dr. S. P. Dey has given a detail of a case of tuberculosis of glands in his work Clinical Case Reports on Constitutional Prescribing, published by Books and Allied (P) Ltd., Kolkata.

Dr Dey writes that his patient was a married lady who was having a left axilla swelling enlarged, malted and suppurated gland. This gland later on showed no sign of cure, even after traditional allopathic treatment. Dr. Dey took the whole history of the patient and prescribed her Streptomycin sulphate and Bacillinum and Chinnum ars. The whole history can be seen in the above referred work of Dr. Dey.

Within one year, the case was cured and gland was healed after discharge of some pus.

Comments : Dr Dey had used Streptomycin (a tautopathic drug). Because the case was over-dosed by allopathic physician, to remove the effects of this drug, he prescribed this medicine in a homoeopathic way and, when the case opened classical homoeopathic medicines cured the case.

Dr. Dey had used all homoeopathic medicines in fifty millesimal scale potency to save the patient's health from any undue aggravation. LM (fifty millesimal scale) potency medicines work faster and safer. Hahnemannian opinion regarding use of this potency scale must be encouraged, specially in those case where the case has some specific sensitivity to particular aliments.

Tautopathy – which has been made popular in India by most respected stalwart. Dr. R. P Patel — should be given a due respect in all those cases which have a dense history of heavy allopathic drugging. The iatrogenic diseases in any cases may be unlocked by the initial use of tautopathic medicines.

Case 6 : Tuberculosis of Bone)

Dr. P. S. Kamthan, a senior physician, has noted a case of tuberculosis of bone in his work Remedies for Skin and Bone Diseases, published by B. Jain Publishers, New Delhi. His patient was a married lady who was suffering from "bone tuberculosis–ulceration of spine in the lumbar region diverting its course to discharge through a brain abscess".

Dr. Kamthan started his treatment by giving her Bacillinum 1M. Then he prescribed Silicea 3X altered with Calcarea sulph 3X. In one year Dr. Kamthan cured the case.

Comments : This case shows that the homoeopathic medicines worked well in a destructive tuberculosis case. As usual, nosode was in high potency and the remaining medicines in low potency; pathology usually requires low potency medicines, provided vital force is strong enough.

Case 7 : (Tuberculosis of intestines)

Most respected and senior physician and propounder of LM potency scale in India, Dr. R. P. Patel, has noted his clinical experience in a case of Tabes-mesentrica (Consumption of bowels).

His patient was a boy having pain (severe) in abdomen, going from right to left, restless, exhausted after pains and unconscious during pain. He was also suffering from headache. He had received allopathic drug stsreptomycin and other drugs.

Dr. R. P. Patel prescribed his patient Nux-vomica, Sulphur, in 0/30 potency, Tuberculinum in 200 potincy and Arnica in 0/6 potency. Dr Patel has written that the case was cured and the homoeopathic medicines treated patient fastly.

Comments : This was a case which was solved by LM potency scale. LM potency scale has got many benefits over traditional potency scales. This scale can be repeated frequently, however, in this case, Dr. Patel had not made so much repetition of medicines. Readers will find that the medicines mostly affecting the G.I.T. have cured the case of tuberculosis (?). Arnica was given due to injury on the abdomen.

The complete detail of the case can be read from Dr. R. P. Patel's work "My Experiments with 50 millesimal Scale Potencies" published by Hahnemann Homoeopathic Pharmacy, Kottayam, Kerala. In the same work, Dr. Patel has noted that he has treated cases of ***tuberculosis of intestines, tubercular glands, tuberculous spine*** and ***tubercular minor leprosy*** — all the cases were relieved. The cases of tubercular glands were cured fully.

N.B. A well-reputed and genius homoeopathist of India, Dr. Sarabhai, has given a list of homoeopathic medicines in affection of tuberculosis in different organs. A detail can be read from his work. Homoeopathic Reminiscence, published by Sarabhai Homoeopathic Foundation, Mumbai.

Medicine	Tuberculosis
Drosera	of bones and glands
Silica	For all diseases of bones including tubercle tendency
Symphytum	Necrotic character of bone situation met in tuberculosis)
Sulphur	Scrofula
Iodium	of glands
Bromium	of glands (enlargement of glands)
Phosphorus	Pulmonary tuberculosis and glandular tuberculosis
Baryta Carb	of gland and bones
Mercury	of bones where abscess has been formed
Theridion	Tubercular diathesis
Cistus Can	Scrofolous child and affection of glands
Tuberculinum	Tubercular susceptibilities develop resistance against tuberculosis

Dr Sarabhai has written that the above medicines are "similie" to disease pattern; but for doing much better the individualization of case is must in any case of tuberculosis.

Case 8 : There are some cases which have been reported by Temple. S. Hoyne in his work "Clinical Therapeutics" Vol. I/II, Published by B. Jain Publishers, New Delhi.

Here the treated tuberculosis and medicines will be indicated. A detailed description may be read from the above source :

Ambra	Pulmonary tuberculosis	When expectoration is yellowish or whitigh, great nervousness and talking
Ammonium muriaticum	Pulmonary tuberculosis	When coldness is felt between scapulas
Antims Tart	Pulmonary tuberculosis	Blood spitting cough, dyspnoea and palpitation, heavy inflammation

Asarum	Pulmonary tuberculosis	Chilly person, short hacking cough, profuse expectoration, stitches in both lungs
Bromine	Phthisis commencing from Vocal cords (tuberculosis of lungs)	Larynx painful, inflamed and ulcerated
Drosera	Pulmonary tuberculosis	Constant chill and cough
Kreosote	Pulmonary tuberculosis	Fever and cough, Vomiting, loss of hunger, stitches in left chest
Stannum	Laryngeal and Tracheal phthisis	Constant short and hacking cough, night sweats

[Some medicines and tuberculosis treatment from Vol. I of T. S. Hoyne's Clinical Therapeutics]

Arsenic	Tuberculosis of Intestines	Repid sinking, emaciation, despairs of life, complains about everything
Nitric Acid	Tuberculosis of Intestines	When most violent cutting pain lasts for a long time in stools, especially in diarrhoea (Acute or Chronic case)

[Some medicines and tuberculosis treatment from Vol. 2 of T. S. Hoyne's Clinical Therapeutics]

Comments : All the referred remedies are age-old classical medicines, their utility is highly beneficial in different forms of tuberculosis.

BIBLIOGRAPHY

Allen H. C. : The Materia Medica of the Nosodes with proving of the X-ray, (B. Jain/New Dehli)

Agrawal Y. R. : A Comparative Study of Chronic Miasms (Vijay publica/ Delhi)

Boericke : Pocket Manual of Homoeopathic Materia Medica and Reportory (B. Jain Publishers/New Delhi)

Burt W. H. : Therapeutics of Tuberculosis (B. Jain Publishers/New Delhi)

Banerjee : A Text Book of Homoeopathic Pharmacy Vol. I/II, B. Jain Publishers/New Delhi

Chand Deewan H.C. : Microdose Megaresut, National Homoeopathic Pharm. New Delhi.

Clarke : Dictionary of Practical Materia Medica Vol. I, II, III, (B. Jain Publishers/New Delhi)

Choudhury. H. : Indications of Miasms (B. Jain Publishers/New Delhi)

Close, Stuart : The Genius of Homoeopathy (I B P P/New Delhi)

Christian H. A. : Principles And Practice of Medicine (D. Appleton Century, London)

Dey, S. P. : Clinical Case Reports on Clinical Prescribing (New Central Book Agency, Kolkata)

Davidson. S. : The Principles and Practice of Medicine (E. L. B. S. publication)

Hahnemann. S. : Chronic Diseases Vols. I/II (I. B. P. P./New Delhi)

Heat F. R. G. : Symposium of Tuberculosis (Casell and Company Ltd. London)

Hoyne Temple : Clinical Therapeutics (2 Vols set) (B. Jain Publishers/New Delhi)

Jullian O. A. : Materia Medica of Nosodes with Reportory — Dictionary of Homoeopathic M. M. (B. Jain Publishers/New Delhi)

Mathur K. N. : Principles of Prescribing (B. Jain Publishers/New Delhi)

Murphy Robin : Homoeopathic Remedy Guide (I B P P/New Delhi)

Murphy Robin : Homoeopathic Medical Repertory (I B P P/New Delhi)

Sarkar. B. K. : Organon of Medicine by Samuel Hahnemann. (M. Bhattacharya & Co., Kolkata)

Sexena Rajeev : A Study of Sarcodes (I B P P/New Delhi)

Saxena Rajeev : A Phenomenological Study of Nosode (B. Jain Publishers/ New Delhi)

Saxena Rajeev : Understanding Glands, Endocrinology, The Homoeopathic Treatment (B. Jain Publishers/New Delhi)

Schroyens F. : Synthesis Reportorium Homoeopathicum Syntheticum (Homoeopathic Book Publishers, London)
Scot Ronald Bodly : Practice of Medicine (E L B S Oxford, London)
Varma & Indu : Encyclopaedia of Homoeopathic Pharmacopoeia Vols. I/II, (B. Jain Publishers/New Delhi)

Journals

Advent of Homoeopathy :
Homoeopathic Heritage:
Homoeo Gagan (Hindi):
National Journal of Homoeopathy